I0123467

Doing a
180
at
60

You-Turn Allowed

John R. Takacs

Red Engine Press
Pittsburgh, Pennsylvania

Library of Congress Control Number: 2016959523

ISBN: 978-1-943267-21-7

Cover design: Joyce Faulkner

Editing: Betsy Beard

Printed in the United States.

Red Engine Press

Dedication

This book is dedicated
to those who never had the privilege
of making it to sixty years of age.

1

The Dream

I. Was. Wrong.

Okay, I admit it. If I had uttered those three words earlier, I could have avoided a lifetime of ignorance.

Now just so you know, I'm not overloaded with ego. I admit to being wrong many times. However, this for me was the BIG wrong. It was the result of believing a lie, one that many of us are guilty of believing. But before I explain, let me first give you a little background.

I was born April 29, 1951, right smack in the middle of the baby boomer years. In our household, I was number five, with three older sisters and an older brother. Then later on there were two younger sisters. Seven of us, in all.

On April 29, 2011, I turned sixty years old. On that fateful day (and I'm sure if you are over thirty you've heard something like this) I was told, "You're not only over the hill…it's more like you're passing through the rusty gates to Boot Hill."

Or how about this one? "Happy birthday, Old Man. You look pretty good," and here comes the zinger, "for your age."

You see, therein lies the problem. My mind doesn't feel any different than it did when I was in my thirties. Sure, I'm a little bit wiser now, but I'm still subject to a screw-up every once in a while.

Before my 60th birthday arrived in 2011, that winter had been a cold one, even for California. It was February, and it was snowing where I lived, up in the mountains. I had just finished writing my second novel, a sequel to my first award-winning novel, *The Take-Us*, and was blissfully content inside my head. At least I thought I was content. However, when I glanced down, I couldn't help but see my stomach hanging over my belt.

Every year for the previous dozen years or so I would start my new "I'm sure it's gonna work this time" diet on New Year's Day. And you know, I *almost* started it that year on New Year's Day 2011.

But, nope! Not that year. Instead, I just decided to be old…and overly fat. You never heard of the term, overly fat? Probably because it's a phrase I've coined.

Since the skinniest of us still have many pounds of body fat, the rest of us have a hefty excess. Hence the term: overly fat. I didn't know it at the time, but I was lugging about sixty pounds of fat. No wonder my feet, knees, and hips hurt, all of which I had been attributing to age.

I stayed overly fat for a few more weeks, from that day in February until the beginning of Lent. I'm Catholic, which is probably not much of a surprise to you since you just read that there were seven kids in my family. But truly, I'm not a very good Catholic, and God knows I'm not being humble.

I've learned many things in life, and one of them is that once a habit is made, it sticks around until a stronger habit breaks it. I had lost the habit of going to church regularly and blamed it on the necessary evil of being on the road promoting my first novel. I was away from home more than I was home in the preceding two and a half years. So when I returned to church, I decided I needed more C—as in Christ—in my life. And since it was the beginning of Lent, I gave up some other Cs, like Candy, Chocolate, Cake, Cookies, Chips, Crackers, and Cream—ice cream, sour cream, sweet creamy butter, the cream in milk, and cheese. Oh, and I gave up the biggest C of them all: Coors.

Doing a 180 at 60

In my own little world, I created the Seven Cs diet. Just for forty days.

It couldn't be that hard, right?

After a few days on my Seven Cs diet, it hit me like a ton of tacos. I was an addict. Well, not a heroin addict, an alcoholic, or a three-pack-a-day smoker, but I was an addict nonetheless—addicted to junk food. An addict is an addict, and short of running to the store for a Snickers bar, I had no clue what to do.

Since I was giving all this up for Lent and the good Lord, I said a prayer. Lo and behold, a miracle occurred. Maybe in the great scheme of things it wasn't an earth-shattering miracle, but for me the cravings stopped. Okay, it could have been that my blood sugar finally reached a normal level and I almost felt human again. Or it could have been that my brain was adjusting to the new regime. But it felt like a miracle, and after all, I had prayed. Of course, at the time I didn't know there were going to be strings attached to the answer. You know, small things.

Like changing my whole life!

Two weeks later, I stepped on the scales and discovered I had lost six pounds. I was still eating well, and all I did was cut out some crap. Believe it or not, by this time I didn't even realize I was on a diet.

Have you ever heard that old saying, "Be careful what you pray for?"

Two months later, a month before my sixtieth birthday, four things happened. The first occurred as I was sitting in the bar after a game of golf with some of the guys who play together regularly. As older men do, we were recalling our youthful adventures and telling stories.

Lots of stories...

I've noticed over the years that the guys who played it pretty straight, worked a lot, and raised families don't seem to have as many stories as those who lived a somewhat *wilder* life. I'm not being judgmental here, but it's a sad thing to get older and have no stories to tell. Now myself, I have lots of stories. So many that I sometimes wonder if my friends think I'm making stuff up. Sometimes I even wonder how I crammed so much in and still managed to work like a dog most of my life. But here's the really cool thing, the first of the four things that happened: I realized that we can still build some truly great stories after the age of sixty. Just keep reading and you'll see what I mean.

The second thing that happened was that I joined the gym. Yeah, I know they don't call them gyms anymore. Now it's a health club or a fitness center, a hoity-toity name for a place you go to and pay to sweat. I hadn't been to a workout joint for many a year, maybe thirty years.

The third thing that happened was I went online and researched a series of websites to try and understand how weight loss really does work. Seriously, rocket science might be easier to understand. Even though I was in the throes of my Seven Cs diet, I still signed up for a twelve-week course, which—in perfect hindsight—I would never, ever recommend, even to my worst enemy. It reinforced for me why I've never been what you might call a joiner. (There is a chapter coming up on weight loss and all the accompanying misery—kind of like a horror story in the middle of this book.) However, the good part of this first attempt was that it paved the way for the fourth item. It gave me a vision. Truly, through all of my travails, I'd never had The Dream before.

The fourth thing, of course, was The Dream.

But first, have you ever noticed that a journey of a thousand miles always begins with…uh-huh…shoe selection? And for me, it went something like this.

"Honey, you need to clean all of those shoes you don't wear anymore out of the hall closet."

Oh, the injusticeof it all: an unexpected, sudden honey-do. But there is now no doubt about it. Closets hold great secrets.

There were motorcycle riding boots and racing boots and golf shoes. Football, soccer, and baseball shoes. Hiking boots and skiing boots. Even my favorite running shoes. I hadn't worn them in such a long time it looked like the shoe strings were rotting. With drooping shoulders and hanging head, I wondered how I could part with those. Then it occurred to me to wonder if maybe I could do any of that stuff again. Okay, sure I hadn't raced or skied or done a lot of the things I used to do fervently for a very long time. And that's what led to The Dream.

Remember at the beginning I stated flat out that I was wrong? So what was I wrong about? Only my entire life philosophy. It was built on a lie.

In 1971, when I was twenty years old, I was in the hospital with plenty of time to think. I had just returned from Vietnam and had stared death in the eye. But that story is in an upcoming chapter, so just hang on. Anyway, back then I stated aloud what would become my major life philosophy.

"You need to do lots of things when you're young, because when you get old, you won't be able to do them."

Doing a 180 at 60

I then proceeded to live my life according to my erroneous life philosophy. You have a life philosophy, too, even if you've never stated it aloud. It's how you've lived your life to this point. Now think about it. Mine sounded about right, you agree? Many of us have fallen for this.

"Do it while you're young."

"You're only young once."

Maybe *The Young and the Restless* even comes into play, although it seems many of the older men I know are so restless they can't sleep through the night any longer. And the only race anymore is to the bathroom.

Speaking of racing, I raced everything I could lay hands on while I was young, including my own legs. In addition, I went flying, skydiving, and diving—as in scuba diving and diving off bridges (with a bungee cord or without one), and diving for abalones in the frigid shark-infested waters off the Northern California coast. I did many of the more common things, too, like tennis, football, and skiing. And let's not forget yoga, dancing, and horse stuff. Altogether, I engaged in more than sixty sports, activities, and adventures.

When I was young I never bothered to write down a bucket list. I was one of those "Just do it" people. Having lived a life of exhilaration, I have come to realize that your past and, perhaps more importantly, your past activities are somewhat like your finger-prints, unique to you. In fact, if you add up all the really cool things you've done throughout your life, you can pretty much tell if you were a ho-hum joiner or a wild-eyed individualist.

But back to my philosophy, how about a moment of clarity here. Was I wrong? Does life as we knew and loved it end at twenty-nine, thirty-five, forty? Stop and think about it, then write down the age when it ended for you.

So what is The Dream, the asked-for prayer? Simply stated, I realized that life wasn't over and that maybe I could revisit the activities and sports of my youth. And not just do these things again, but improve upon them: beat my times, go higher, go farther, go longer, go deeper, and enjoy it!

The title of this book is *Doing a 180 at 60.* "Doing a 180" is a term for reversing direction, going the opposite way, a U-turn. That is what I needed to do with my life in order to redo, or at least try to do, many of the things I had enjoyed in my life to this point.

I understood perfectly how difficult this was going to be. After all, I was going to try to better some of those previously accomplished goals.

Someone always has to go first. I am that person.

Doing a 180 at 60

And here's where you come into the picture. If I can redo the things I did when I was younger, maybe you can work your way into decent shape and be able to do the things you enjoyed, too. Just think of the stories you can build.

We've all heard the expression, "You're only as old as you feel." The problem is we all have bad days, days we feel like a walking fossil. There are some days that it takes all of our willpower just to get out the door. What a surprise when I tell you it's your body that leads the march and drags your mind out of the gutter, not vice versa.

So hang on and buckle up. I think you're really going to like this trip.

If you wrote down an age, I hope you did it in pencil, because the ride truly starts, not ends, at sixty.

Sixty is the youth of old age.

180 AT 60 REDO LIST

- ☐ Scuba Diving
- ☐ Long Bicycle Tour
- ☐ Golfing
- ☐ Skydiving
- ☐ Flying
- ☐ Motorcycle Tour
- ☐ Abalone Diving
- ☐ Water Skiing
- ☐ Snow Skiing
- ☐ Day Hiking
- ☐ Dirt Bike Riding
- ☐ Racquetball
- ☐ Basketball
- ☐ Baseball
- ☐ Football
- ☐ Tennis
- ☐ Ping Pong
- ☐ Bowling
- ☐ Pool
- ☐ Horseshoes
- ☐ Snowmobiling
- ☐ Jet Skiing
- ☐ Canoeing
- ☐ Kayaking
- ☐ Whitewater Rafting
- ☐ Diving off Rocks
- ☐ Diving off Rope Swing
- ☐ Triathlon
- ☐ Wake Board
- ☐ Run a Marathon

- ☐ Swim One Mile
- ☐ Fishing
- ☐ Skeet Shooting
- ☐ Weightlifting
- ☐ Volleyball
- ☐ Croquet
- ☐ Badminton
- ☐ Horseback Riding
- ☐ Bungee Jumping
- ☐ Zip Line
- ☐ Rappelling
- ☐ Roller Skating
- ☐ Inline Skating
- ☐ Ice Skating
- ☐ Hockey
- ☐ Spelunking
- ☐ Pole Vaulting
- ☐ High Jumping
- ☐ Karate
- ☐ Dancing
- ☐ Soccer
- ☐ Snowshoeing
- ☐ Handball
- ☐ Yoga
- ☐ Archery
- ☐ Trampoline
- ☐ Backpacking
- ☐ Rock Climbing
- ☐ Mountain Biking
- ☐ Write Nonfiction Book

2

Davy Jones's Locker

The first time I went scuba diving I was about ten years old. I grew up in Northern Indiana and lived about a quarter mile from the Saint Joseph River. The river depth varies from twelve feet to twenty-plus feet when you get past the shallows along the banks. There is a golf course there which the river runs through, and you have to hit your golf ball across that river in three different places. Something about hitting the ball over water freaks out even good golfers, and many splash their balls into the water. A few of the holes also border the river, and wayward golf balls occasionally find themselves in the drink.

My mom said that golf was a rich man's sport, so all summer long I made it my job to find and sell the good golf balls back to the rich golfers. One summer, must have been around 1961, my brother Don (two years older) and I decided to buy a scuba tank and regulator. Or I could have written that my brother talked me into going half, because I had no clue. We weren't buying the diving gear for the fun of it, but as a business investment—uh-huh. If you can remember Mike Nelson (Lloyd Bridges) in the TV show *Sea Hunt*, you'll know what kind of equipment we bought.

Things were a bit different back then. (You may see those words again.) No certification, no parental consent, and no release of liability were required for the sale, just cold cash. When we asked how to "do scuba diving," the guy behind the counter said, "Just breathe with your mouth and pop your ears once in a while."

"Heck," I thought, "I can do that!" Never mind that I had no clue what popping your ears meant. My brother and I got the tank full of air, and then he put it on his back and rode his bicycle, Old Betsy, to the river. I carried everything else and showed up at the river with a bunch of friends in tow. It was the height of the baby boom years, and there were lots of kids our age. And after all, this was now the main event in the neighborhood. I'm sure you can imagine it. We were diving to golf ball heaven where we would gather golf balls, like pearls off the ocean floor, and become rich.

My brother dove first, and after about half an hour, it was my turn. Try to picture this. I was a short, skinny kid, and the scuba tank was almost the same height as I was. I was maybe twelve inches taller. So after a bunch of adjustments, I got the tank on and got ready to get in the water. My brother, in a great fit of pure genius, realized we had a small problem. Namely, that I couldn't swim. No big deal. He just tied a rope around my waist and I got into the water.

I kicked and kicked and used my arms like big old paddles, but to no avail. No matter how I kept trying to dive down, I kept popping up. The air in the tank was too buoyant, and I wasn't heavy enough to sink. Most of us kids would go fishing all of the time, and we knew we needed sinkers to get the bait to sink down to the bottom. Yep, the bait was just fine with my big brother tying some bricks around my waist. Down I went into the murky water, fascinated, but only for a moment. After all, I was now a professional diver, and somewhere on the river bottom a huge cache of balls waited to make me rich beyond my greatest dreams.

I had balls to find, never realizing of course, I had already found them.

My parents never had a clue we were diving the "treacherous river full of undertows and currents" (their words). Later on that summer when I asked my mom if I could take swimming lessons, I got kudos for being so mature for my age.

I went on to buy a set of twin tanks and a modern single-hose regulator and dove each summer, until I discovered girls or something else equally destructive.

As a side note, I never had an allowance and paid for everything I owned with my own money, made on the golf course. I never realized until much later that some days I made as much selling used golf balls as my dad did working in the brewery all day.

* * *

Remember that my basic idea was to repeat or try to redo things I'd done in my past, maybe improving upon some of them. When I first jotted down the list of all the things I'd done, they were in no particular order. At least that's what I told myself. However, the truth is that a few days after my sixtieth birthday, we were off to Mexico for a week.

You know how you always want to look good in a bathing suit? Yes, even at sixty. The worst thing that can happen on your holiday is to be harpooned on the beach, mistaken for a whale. I had lost a lot of weight by now—yippee—and I know you're just dying to know about this, so I'll go into it in depth in following chapters.

One week before the trip to Mexico, I decided I wanted to get my scuba certification, which just happened to be the first thing on my redo list. I guess one thing you need to know about me is I'm really good at putting things off until the last minute. I mean, why plan all this stuff out if the world suddenly comes to an end and you wasted all of your time planning instead of living? Yeah…my sweetie didn't go for that one either.

Anyway, I went online and, after a little research, found the Professional Association of Diving Instructors (PADI) website. It cost me $120 to sign up, and I crammed to finish the book-learning part the day before we left for Mexico. That way I could relax on vacation instead of studying.

Off the coast of Mexico is a place called Isla Mujeres. It's a small island in the Caribbean Sea, eight miles off the coast of Cancun. It is a cool place that's really not on the tourist trap map. Not yet commercialized in a big way, it has a quaint feel about it that's hard to describe. Everyone who was on our trip wants to keep it secret, unspoiled—you know, selfish-like. It has a main street with many good restaurants and fun stuff going on, like bars, booze, and cantinas stuffed full of food not allowed on my Seven Cs diet plan.

Doing a 180 at 60

I was in training, so I decided to go to bed early our first night there. After ten or so (lost count) margaritas' and a Cuban cigar (although really, I don't smoke) I accomplished my goal and got to bed early, meaning the very early hours of the morning. Wisdom dictates that at this point in life when you've done nothing but work out for months, you should tape your mouth shut and definitely not eat from a straw your first night out. You should be eating healthy food. Of course, if limes are considered food, I kind of did that.

The next morning I awoke with my head pounding and my mouth feeling like my tongue was scraped against a cactus all night long. After a quart of Joe, I slipped on my bathing suit and walked about a hundred feet to the prettiest beach I've never seen. The sun was so bright and my nicotine-stained eyes so squinted, that I stumbled to a lounge chair and collapsed.

You're probably thinking, "He fell asleep in the sun and got a horrible sunburn."

Hey, I'm no rookie here. I got an umbrella and fell asleep in the shade. But the sun was so intense reflecting off the pure white sand, that I woke up with a horrible sunburn. Of course, it was only on the half of my body facing the sun, making me look like a half-cooked lobster.

It was in between naps that I discovered Sol from one of those nice men that kept walking by. They were carrying big buckets of ice cold beer with the name of Sol, which technically didn't start with the letter C. Later that night I found out Sol translated from Spanish into the word sun. I believe I also found that out in the cold shower, trying to cool off (no not that) my inner and outer sunburn. I know this book is about redoing, and this isn't the kind I'm referring to, but every time I go to Mexico it seems I redo some rendition of the night described above.

The following day I resumed my somewhat foggy training schedule, beginning with a vigorous walk in the perfectly warm morning sun. Ah, life is good the day *after* the day after.

Isla Mujeres is about three and a half miles long, and I walked half way down it, by the way, in perfect safety. I went to a local dive shop, Scuba Adventures, where I had made an appointment. Once there I met Manuel, my Master Diver scuba instructor. He spent many years in the United States and spoke English better than me [Editor's Note: better than I].

I've had many, many instructors in my life, and without a doubt Manuel is the best ever, patient beyond reason. Since all communication underwater is with hand signals, every time he spoke while on land he would use his hands in addition to his calm and sing-song way of speaking. By the time we were in the water, I had all the signals down pat. Manuel was professional and competent, and not one time did I ever feel he didn't have the answer or, maybe more importantly, that I was in any danger.

Manuel and I started in the swimming pool, and he was surprised at how comfortable I was taking the regulator in and out of my mouth and taking the mask off underwater. If he'd ever been in the Saint Joseph River and had a submerged tree branch rip off his mask, he would not have been surprised at all. He told me it was scary how quickly I learned, and I believe he was waiting to be pinched to see if I was for real.

The problem was that when they asked me online if I had ever been certified to dive, I answered no. There wasn't a place on the form to tell them that I probably had 100 or more dives to my credit.

Later that day and the next, we completed my five regulation dives, and all were exactly the same as well as totally different, if you know what I mean. I had graduated from the murky water of the river to the almost perfect clarity of the Caribbean.

Much has been written about the beauty, stunning colors, and serenity of life underwater, so I won't go into that. For me, the quiet is what I noticed more than anything. It was just me and my breathing, kind of what the guy at the scuba shop had told me fifty years before.

After the fifth dive, I had to take all my gear off except my weight belt and float in the Caribbean for a half hour with white caps breaking over my head, and I loved it. When I emerged, I received my certificate as an Open Water Scuba Diver.

My first redo was complete, and I was now certified to dive, something I had never attained in my younger days.

* * *

I have five sisters but only one brother. Don was always taller, could run faster, and jump higher. And of course, he was smarter. He taught me much about all, even how to survive and live through the Vietnam War. He was drafted and fought there the year before I did, and we both served with the famed 101st Airborne Division. All through my youth, I was Don's shadow and he was my hero. I loved him much.

He died in 1995 at the age of forty-six. He had cancer, a type listed by the Department of Veterans Affairs as being caused by Agent Orange. I guess if you think about it, he was killed in the Vietnam War; it just took him twenty-five years to die.

He never made it to sixty.

3

Bicycling

"Just like riding a bicycle. Once you do it, you'll never forget."

Do you remember the first time you rode a bicycle—not a tricycle, but a bicycle—after the training wheels came off? I do. I've noticed when there is a strong emotional response like pain, memories last a long time and are crystal clear.

I was five, and I leaned the bike next to the porch so I could climb on. Off I went up the drive, swung around, and soon was barreling down the driveway pointed directly toward the garage. We had double doors on the garage and a rose bush growing between them on a trellis. It's been more than fifty-five years, and this is still painful to recall.

Apparently there was an international bicycle brake recall for which we never got the memo. Can

Doing a 180 at 60

you think of any other reason why, on my first solo bike ride, I crashed into the rose bush, thereby becoming a human pin cushion? Apparently, back in those days, we just took personal responsibility and never sued the bike manufacturer for not putting a sticker on the bike warning that rose bushes can be hazardous to your health. My mom dusted me off, and a few tears and a cookie or two later, I got back on the bike. To this day, I have never crashed into another rose bush. Yet!

We lived out in the country then—now it's the suburbs—and we had no bus service, so bicycling or hoofing it was the only way to get around. As a kid I rode everywhere and enjoyed it most of the time. Like everybody else back then, when I turned sixteen and got my driver's license, my bike riding days were over.

I really didn't ride again until my late twenties when I bought a new bike, a French Motobécane ten-speed. Since I took French in high school, I figured it was meant to be. It was supposed to be for therapy to help a damaged knee (details in an upcoming chapter). But it was stolen a few months later from in front of the home of a doctor friend of mine who lived in a great neighborhood. I assumed it was my fault since I got a C in French and didn't remember the word for "lock."

After I moved to California, my good friend and running partner Davey called me up one sunny day and told me to bring my checkbook. He informed me we were going to start riding bicycles together, since it was easier on our bodies than running. I was thirty-four at the time, and after spending way too much, I was the proud owner of an aluminum Trek 1500, twelve-speed, skinny-tire, road bike—American made (I had much better grades in English).

I cannot even begin to tell you how hooked I became on bicycle riding. Many nights after work and on weekends, we would ride from San Jose, over the pass at Mount Madonna, and down to Santa Cruz. We'd have a beer on the wharf and then ride back over the mountains, doing about a hundred miles, roundtrip.

It was on those first rides that I discovered the secret to long, difficult ascents over mountain passes. When you can see the top of the mountain, some unknown reservoir of energy comes up from below to give you the strength and power to climb over the top. It's the unknown that make things so difficult. The secret is to lie to yourself and keep telling yourself, "I think the top is just past this approaching corner." I know this may sound weird, but eventually you'll come around that last corner for real and see the top of the mountain. A quick burst of energy suddenly fills you, and you're over the top.

Once you get over, you can coast—and even scream—down the other side, soon forgetting the pain. This same technique works for many other difficult times in life. After all, the bicycle saying, "Once one hill ends, another begins," is a constant throughout life.

A month before I turned sixty, I was riding my exercise bike upstairs, sweating like a pig, mostly because I was way overweight. Let me clarify that word usage. According to the government weight chart, I've been overweight since I was seventeen. I don't have big bones, but I did have some muscle mass, kind of like football players. They are all overweight, but not overly fat. However, now I had the dreaded furniture disease, where my chest had slipped down to my drawers.

The truth was, my muscles had disappeared, and I was really getting overly fat. You ask how I knew that? I got tanked. That is, I was tested for body fat by being submerged in a tank and weighed underwater.

Anyway, I was riding the exercise bike and out of the blue came a memory of a conversation I had with an ex-neighbor in San Jose. She was way older than I was. At the time I was thirty-seven, and she had to have been in her mid-forties. (Hey, when you're younger, it seems that way. Perspective is everything.) She told me she had completed the Davis Double Century one-day bike tour, starting in the wee hours of the morning and finishing about midnight.

I never had the courage to try riding 200 miles in one day when I was younger, but for some odd reason I decided at nearly sixty years old that I wanted to try this. No freaking clue!

I don't know about you, but I have a little voice that pops up in my head occasionally and shouts, "Are you crazy?" Now, some people might think they're going insane when they start hearing voices. However, as a novelist I'm used to hearing dialogue in my mind all day long. Many times I even speak sentences out loud to see if they sound phony before typing them out.

But this time I recognized that particular voice and knew it was me trying to negotiate with me. That's real sanity for you. My head was making a deal with my body, which of course was going to have to do all the work. We all agreed that for me to ride the Davis Double I would have to weigh less than 189 pounds. It was a pretty crafty deal my body cut, seeing as how I weighed 215 pounds and only had about eight weeks to lose almost twenty-five pounds. That would be precisely the same twenty-five pounds I had been trying half-heartedly to lose for the previous ten years.

Doing a 180 at 60

Haven't we all been told how hard it is for us "old" people to lose weight?

At the time, I was riding my Lifecycle exercise bike one hour at a sitting, about sixteen miles. Sizzling with new energy, I doubled my time to two hours and did it every other day. I also joined the f-f-f-fitness center—oh hell, *gym*—and started an online diet. I am not going to go into a lot of the details, but something really magical happened to me, because the weight started dropping off as if an old buzzard was pecking it off. I kept a log of everything I ate and all the exercise I was doing, which is how I started disagreeing with the experts who say weight loss is just diet and exercise.

Diet is pretty easy to understand: get rid of the junk food, eat fewer calories and more high-quality food, and add protein—lots. Although…there is a problem with the definition of high quality food. It seems to have many different meanings for many people, some of whom even have a kind of religious fervor about it.

Exercise is a little easier to understand, maybe. I live across the street from a golf course and love to play. The problem is, no matter how you slice it (and do I ever), golf is not really exercise. It's more of an activity. In order to be considered exercise, you must perform at your target heart rate—beats per minute (bpm)—and be able to sustain it for a while. According to some experts' current research, the long slow exercise regime is not nearly as effective as high intensity interval training (HIIT). There's more on this in upcoming chapters.

How do you get a heart rate zone established? It goes something like this. First subtract your age from 220 and multiply the result by 65% for fat burn or 80% for aerobic. For me, that translated to: 220 minus 60 equals 160, times 80% for a target heart rate of 128 bpm. The more accurate Karvonen Method is more complicated and factors in resting heart rate to calculate target heart rate. However, until you really get involved in an exercise program, the simple calculation is close enough. Like almost everything else in life, this is a guide and not written in stone.

When golfing, I very seldom ride in a golf cart. Most of the time I walk the course—four and a half miles around and back to my house. If I were exercising, I would need to walk that distance in less than an hour. Playing golf takes four hours or more, so it's clearly not getting my heart rate up. But it is *movement*, and that's the third rail of weight loss, especially since four hours of moving about and swinging once in awhile keeps me away from food.

Doing a 180 at 60

My exercise regime began to settle into this: every day I would walk my dog Sam for an hour, which equals more movement. The weather was lousy that spring and I was having trouble getting three rounds of golf per week. (Do I hear violins for my pity party?) Even if I played golf every other day, I would still go to the gym, do the elliptical machine, core work, and weight lifting, finishing with a swim. On the other day I would ride my exercise bike for two hours. I would take off one day a week for recovery, usually Sunday. (I wonder where I got that concept.) An easy day always followed a hard day.

This concept was one of the most difficult things for me to figure out and do. I wanted to work, work, work. However, it's the rest that allows my body to rebuild and get stronger. There is a term for what I do, and it's called active recovery.

A couple weeks before my sixtieth birthday, it occurred to me that if I was going to ride the double century, I had a small problem. And that was that I needed to get on a real bike and ride. I convinced myself it wasn't a big deal and finally got my dusty and trusty twenty-six-year-old Trek off the hangers in the garage. Luckily, it was an aluminum bike. Otherwise it would have been rusty. It was amazing to me that my bicycle was twenty-six years old. It seemed like only yesterday.

I loaded the bicycle into my car and drove it down to my local shop to be tuned up, replacing a few things like the cycling computer, cables, tubes, and rotting tires. One day later, I loaded the bike into the back of my car and drove down to the American River Bike Trail in Sacramento, only sixty-five miles away.

The trail is about thirty-three miles long and runs from Folsom Lake Dam to Discovery Park in downtown Sacramento. It was a perfect place to practice without having to worry about automobile traffic, especially since I was a tad nervous from such a long bicycling hiatus.

As a side note, one of the main ideas in my redo plan is to keep from spending a fortune on new equipment. Keep the costs down and use what you have where practicable. (Okay, so I'm a bit thrifty, which is a nice way of saying I'm cheap.)

I began riding my skinny-wheeled bike for the first time in sixteen years. I rode for more than three hours, covering fifty-one miles on my first time out and finished… exhausted. Four days later it was sixty-four miles, and then the day before my birthday, I rode eighty-three miles. For the first time, I allowed the top of the mountain to slip into my head, thinking how difficult it was going to be…and I hadn't even ridden half the distance yet.

Three days later, I made it to the midway point and rode 100.3 miles in six hours and fifty-two minutes. The following day I got on a plane for my Mexico scuba adventure.

While in Mexico, it did occur to me that I hadn't had enough time to build the endurance for such a long excruciating ride. In fact, all of the experts were telling me that it's not possible to lose weight so fast *and* build endurance at the same time.

But wait a minute there, Hoss. I know that's not true, because I'd seen overly fat guys in basic training do it. Maybe you're thinking, "Yeah, and they were eighteen years old." But you just read how in two weeks I went from riding zero miles to one hundred, so maybe it isn't only about age.

When I got back from Mexico, I went for a few more rides, fifty milers, while testing different seats (because even though my legs were getting strong, my crotch was sore). Then at sixty years and two weeks, I rode 127.6 miles. I had one week left before the big ride. The following day I weighed 189.5 pounds. Oh, crap. Since my goal was to be less than 190, I had no excuse for backing out now.

Luck almost always plays a part in a great achieve-
ment. What was lucky for me was going to Mexico
and not being able to train for a week. It forced me
to rest and recover. I didn't realize how I had over-
strained and overtrained.

I'm used to getting up around six in the morning,
but I began practicing getting up at three for the final
two weeks so when the day arrived I wouldn't be
shocking my body so badly. You can see I really live
in a delusional world. Bike 200 miles in a day and
not shock my body? But seriously, I had a strategy. I
knew that if I could hang on and make it to the 150
mile marker, I'd be too stubborn to quit even if I had
body parts falling off. Also, as I taught my kids, "Once
the check is written, there is no quittin' period." Told
you I was cheap.

I showed up at the starting line at five o'clock
in the morning and hung around for five minutes,
nervously watching some other riders beginning the
quest. Without any fanfare or fans, at 5:05 on a cool
Saturday morning in Davis, California, I mounted my
faithful steed and began a journey that twenty-five
years previously, I didn't think I could make.

In the first hours I was passed by many riders,
no big deal. These are some of the best conditioned
people in California, and in the bottom of my heart

Doing a 180 at 60

I knew I was not. However, hours later I was passed by three riders—one guy and two girls—going just a bit faster than me. I pushed myself and joined up with them, my legs burning.

I stayed with them until we began climbing up those big mountains that I hadn't even known existed. (I hadn't bothered to read the information the race organizers sent me and somehow assumed it was going to be a flat valley ride. As it turns out, I didn't have time to train for the climbs anyway.) Off they went out of my sight. Did I mention that one of the girls had a prosthetic where her lower leg was missing? I was amazed she could persevere. So much for feeling sorry for myself! In fact, I was glad to have two aching legs.

Cobb Mountain. Does that send shivers up your spine? How about drops of sweat down it? We began climbing many hours before and *seriously* climbing at about mile marker forty. I have come to realize that although two hundred miles is a long way, what really makes it difficult is the amount of climbing you have to do in this ride—more than 8,000 feet of total vertical climbing when you add up every hill.

The top of Cobb Mountain was just past the halfway point, 107 miles. A couple of miles before the top, I had to get off and push my bike. I wasn't the only one. I had been riding at three miles per hour—and now walking even slower—and it didn't take but a few breaths to realize I would never finish the event at such a slow speed. So I dug deep and remounted and grunted away to the top, lying to myself about every corner and the next rest stop.

Speaking of rest stops, there were nine of them spaced out over the ride, and for much of the ride, I fantasized about getting to each of them. You see, my real strategy lies deep within this revelation. A ride of two hundred miles is just too big to comprehend. However, if I can just ride twenty-five miles from one rest stop to another, those little bites make the elephant go down nicely. All the rest stops were well stocked with healthy foods as well as junk food. It was kind of cool to eat as many Oreo's as I wanted and then go burn them off.

I have to put this in here because I am not some kind of super athlete. Hell, I'd never tried anything like this before. I'm just like everyone else in that I hurt and my breath burns and I have all kinds of aches and pains constantly popping up. The difference is that I've learned to negotiate with them. I have a feeling we'll discuss this topic much more throughout the book.

I was wearing my iPod, which I've nicknamed my Walkman, probably because I keep forgetting the word "iPod." When I made mile marker 150 and started a long downhill section, Steely Dan came on, singing "Hey Nineteen." It made me mad when he sang, "She thinks I'm crazy, but I'm just growing old." I used the anger for inspiration for the next mile or so, but got over it pretty quickly. I was getting tired by then, and holding grudges just made it worse.

Darkness fell around nine that night, and by then I'd ridden about 175 miles. I caught up with a guy who was smart enough to have some really powerful lighting (not like me who couldn't see the road ten feet in front of my wheel with my feeble little light). Come to think of it, I can't remember the last time I had ridden a bicycle at night. We rode on and on. It was so different not being able to see around you, and instead it was kind of mesmerizing looking down at the road. I began to get stronger, "smelling" the finish line not too far distant.

At 11:15, exactly eighteen hours and ten minutes after I started, I crossed the finish line. Not being macho or manly or whatever, but I did have enough for a couple more hours. I was tired, but slightly out-of-kilter happy and maybe a little mind numb, which is probably why I thought I could ride a few more hours. Still, I was glad I didn't have to go any farther. I felt strange after I accomplished something so big, not like I wanted to shout, but more like something inside my soul simply settled into place. The almost surreal feeling of inner peace had arrived.

Was I sore? Only everything from my cramped toes to my sunburned ears. And you really don't want to read about my crotch…really.

These are not the official stats, but they are very close. There were 913 total entries, 58 no-shows (but they tell me most of these people ride, just without checking in), and 54 riders who didn't finish. I did finish, after doing everything wrong. (See the results at davisbikeclub.org. I was number 730)

I did something I couldn't do (or at least thought I couldn't do) back when my good friend Davey talked me into bicycle riding so many years ago.

* * *

Davey and I met while working together. He was a really hard worker and extremely resourceful. He was a great guy and a good friend. When he first moved to California, he lived with me. I was in his wedding.

I cried when, at the age of forty-five, he was killed in a car crash on his way to work.

He never made it to sixty.

4

Motorcycle Mania

If it has handlebars, two wheels, a seat, and an engine, is it a motorcycle?

The engine was from a lawnmower, a Briggs and Stratton engine which had a drive shaft that came out the side—not like today's bottom design. The wheels were short and fat. A pulley was attached to the rear wheel, and a fan belt went to the pulley on the engine. In between was a pedal that you pushed down with your left foot. When you pushed down on the pedal, another pulley tightened the belt and away you went. It was great fun until the sheriff showed up and my dad made me sell it. Talk about injustice: I was being labeled a motorcycle gang member at twelve years old.

Maybe it *was* a handmade motor scooter, but it was, for me, the start of a love of two-wheeled motors that is one of the three great adventure loves I have most consistently followed throughout my life.

I bought my first real motorcycle when I was nineteen and home on leave from the Army. It was a Honda 160cc, the same kind of motorcycle Mike, one of my best friends, had and that I had learned to ride on when we were growing up, which means it had a clutch and you had to shift it. In my garage right now I have a Honda HRS216 push lawnmower, with an HVC160 engine. That would be the same size engine that my first motorcycle had. I'm sure you'll understand how much sense it made when I tied a blanket and some clothes behind me (with twine) and attempted to ride from Northern Indiana to Fort Bragg, North Carolina. I had recently graduated from The United States Army Airborne School, and as a new paratrooper I was fearless… or young, dumb, and indestructible.

Before I left Indiana, my dad pushed twenty dollars into my pocket. Added to what money I already had, I now possessed forty-five dollars to go almost a thousand miles. After riding all day through Indiana, I followed a concrete drainage ditch that went up a steep hill in Kentucky and spent the first night in bliss, overlooking the highway and sleeping on the ground next to my motorcycle. I'm telling you, I knew how those cowboys felt lying by the campfire in the Old West, except there wasn't a campfire and I was in the South. It was still very cool. I spent the second night on the ground in Tennessee and arrived the third day at Fort Bragg, ecstatic—albeit with a sore butt (maybe a pattern here).

As I look back at that trip, I wonder how goofy I had to be to ride a thousand miles on a lawnmower engine. That bike got over a hundred miles per gallon, and gas was only about thirty cents a gallon. Can you imagine going a thousand miles on five bucks today? I was eating McDonald hamburgers at nineteen cents a pop and had money left over when I arrived at Fort Bragg.

Beginning with that motorcycle, I have owned thirty-one motorcycles in my life. Most of them have been dirt bikes, but I also have owned the following street motors: Harleys, Kawasakis, Suzukis, Yamahas, BMWs, and more Hondas. I still have five motorcycles, and if I sell one I'll probably buy two others. That would be what one could call a serious addiction.

I live in Northern California and have ridden north to Seattle and south to San Diego. After riding those thousand early miles as a kid, I dreamed (like most motorcyclists) of riding across the country, coast to coast. But every time I would think, dream, or plan it,

Doing a 180 at 60

I never had the time. Or if I had the time, I didn't have the money. Funny how something you decide, something you deem important, just keeps getting pushed to the back of the pack. You'll get to it, but when?

In 1999, at the age of forty-eight, I bought a BMW 1100RT when I thought I had throat cancer. It turned out to be acid reflux, but the reason I bought that bike is that I figured I was going belly-up. Whoa, hypochondriac, you're thinking? Remember, though, my brother had died of cancer just a couple of years before. So don't think I didn't think about it. Maybe I overreacted. However, since I did have a brand-new motorcycle, I thought I would finally achieve my cross-country goal. But I can't say I was disappointed when I found out I would live. Why didn't I go then? Don't know, can't remember, and maybe life just got in the way again.

Ten quick years later in 2009, I won a gold medal for my thriller, *The Take-Us*, from Military Writers Society of America. The award ceremony was scheduled to be in Orlando, Florida, around the first of October. I had the time. I had the money. I even had a legitimate tax write-off. So what was the problem? Oh, Lord, the ugly truth is that I honestly didn't know if I was in good enough shape to go 3,000 miles there and another 3,000 back. It makes you wonder what happened to that guy on the lawnmower engine.

I remember thinking, "You know, I could do it." But then I thought of all of the reasons why I couldn't, like: how can I take some books; and oh, yeah, my suit would get wrinkled; and let's not forget it might rain or snow, or a tsunami might wash Florida away. I also had a speaking engagement scheduled in Sacramento the week before.

Not being able to decide, I asked my sweet girl, lifelong partner and best friend. She said (and this is the bottom-line truth), "If you don't do it now, you might be too old to do it later." And I thought she was right. So I rode from my home to Sacramento, finished speaking, rode to central Florida and back, and was blissfully content with the possible exception of freezing my butt off.

I almost fulfilled the goal. Perhaps you caught my mistake? You see, my cross-country dream was to ride from coast to coast, not from the middle of California to the middle of Florida. Small thing?

Dreams defined become goals, and it was empty because I didn't do it—and worse, I knew it.

So a couple months after I turned sixty, on a foggy Saturday morning in June of 2011, my motorcycle was parked on The Wharf in Santa Cruz, California. There

Doing a 180 at 60

was a car show going on featuring the old woodies (pre-1952 wood-bodied cars), and I was having breakfast as the sun broke through the coastal overcast. I could not have had a better omen.

On Sunday, I was enjoying fresh lobster in a small restaurant at Nauset Beach, Cape Cod, Massachusetts. Oh yeah, that was one week later. It was the accomplishment of accomplishments to finally go all the way from one coast to the other.

I could describe most of that trip in minute detail, but unless you were there, you would miss the fresh smell of the rain and woods, oceans, and plains. You wouldn't experience the feeling of freedom that comes from watching the road seemingly disappear into the side of a mountain in the middle of the desert somewhere in Nevada. It's only as I've aged that I learned to appreciate the fullness of the emptiness of the desert.

Hey, do you think I could be the next Deepak? Maybe not.

I never tired of the sounds of the different types of pavement beneath my tires, transmitting the constant healthy feel of power, generating between my legs and flowing through my hands and ending in my heart.

Dangerous? Well, of course.

I had three close calls, two of them occurring when a driver was texting and drifted into my lane. The other one happened when I was going through Chicago and a little old lady started to cut me off. She had her window down and I yelled, "Hey!" and she veered back into her own lane. All my previous working out must have given me a good set of lungs… or else I was scared and screaming for my life.

I've been cut off many, many times in my life. When I was young, I thought it was deliberate and always had my middle finger loaded and ready. As I got older, I realized most people just don't see a motorcycle in traffic. How do I know that? I did it once myself and found myself kowtowing to the motorcyclist, begging his forgiveness. Meanwhile, he simply hit his brakes, darted around me, and kept on going as I had done a hundred times before.

Something about the open road creates the feeling of freedom, but it wouldn't be right to tell you it's all hunky-dory. Motorcycling is dangerous, and I have had some crashes. Some were on me, some weren't. The dumbest crash happened when I had been drinking. I hit a median about two o'clock in the morning and went down wearing jeans and jacket, receiving a bad case of road rash for my stupidity. The worst, however, was not my fault and occurred way up in the mountains in Yosemite National Park.

I was leaning into a tight curve at about fifty miles per hour when a white car coming from the other direction was in my lane. With only fractions of a second to spare, I had to straighten my motorcycle. Like a matador facing an oncoming bull, I narrowly escaped the car, which brushed past me within inches. I couldn't make the curve, though, and had to lay the motorcycle down.

I got off and away just before the motorcycle went through the brush and off a steep cliff, finishing about eighty feet below the road. For me, it was like a miracle that I collided with some little trees, more like bushes, and they gently laid me down with just a raspberry on my knee and elbow. The worst part was when I walked down the road to see where my motorcycle ended up and noticed I was limping. I didn't feel any pain and then noticed the heel of my right boot was ripped off. I had the one-foot-flat walk going.

This was out in the boonies, and I was really lucky that another motorcycle came along soon after. I flagged him down and told him what happened. It took the park ranger an hour to get to me, and for the last half of the hour I could hear his siren getting closer and closer. He finally arrived and figured I must be in shock when he saw where the motorcycle was. It really was a close call.

* * *

I'm no angel, and I had some wild and crazy times on my motorcycles, like the time I rode my Harley in the back door of the Hi Neighbor Bar in Indianapolis and did a burnout through the bar. My good friend Mike was there that night. It was he who got me started on motorcycles with his Honda 160. He was a giant of a man, at 6'7" and 280 pounds or more, and he loved riding. He really was that guy (when he was single) who parked his Harley in his living room in the middle of winter to work on it.

I will never forget the time he drank too much and I couldn't talk him into staying overnight at my house. He said, with that crooked smile he almost always had on, "I never hit a stationary object in my life," and then proceeded to back his El Camino into a tree in my front yard. I laughed so hard I fell to the ground and he soon joined me.

He was a good friend with a great sense of humor. When he died of a heart defect at the age of forty-eight, life was never the same for me.

He didn't even make sixty.

5

Up in the Air

My dad was a paratrooper in World War II. I was a second-generation jumper at the age of eighteen, having graduated from jump school at Fort Benning, Georgia, in January 1970. My son is also a paratrooper, serving with the 82nd Airborne and has been deployed to Iraq and Afghanistan. He's a third-generation jumper, which is somewhat rare.

So what would make anyone want to jump out of a perfectly good airplane? To begin with, there is no such thing as a perfectly good airplane; every landing is just a controlled crash. Not going for that? How about an extra $55 hazardous duty pay per month? Not yet? How about your dad telling you, "You're not tough enough, and there's no way you can make it." Well, that pretty much cements it.

Doing a 180 at 60

The first week we started jump school was called detail week. Starting on Monday we did all the menial jobs, killing time until everybody showed up. On Friday they gathered us into a giant formation of about a thousand soldiers from all over the world, and the drill instructors took us for a run. The last part of the run was up a hill aptly named Cardiac Hill.

You have to understand the Army to know the run was only a couple of miles, but made more difficult by the instructors constantly screaming at us. "You're not tough enough stuff." At the conclusion of the run, they gathered us into the same giant formation and told us, "If you think that was hard, wait until jump school begins on Monday. If you want to quit, it's okay, because after all, it is voluntary."

To my surprise, about 200 guys quit right then and there. The next day was Saturday, and we repeated the run, extending it a bit farther. The instructors announced the same thing about quitting at the end of the run, and another hundred or so guys quit. All day Sunday the tension was so great you could cut it with a knife, and it wasn't just me. There were a whole lot of nervous guys come Monday morning when jump school officially began.

After our morning formation we started out running, but only went a quarter mile or so before the instructors slowed us down to walk a bit. We all wanted to know what kind of tricks they had up their sleeves. Then we ran just a bit farther than the first time and walked a bit less. And so it went. The drill instructors gradually built us up throughout the weeks of school. Those first runs up Cardiac Hill were just to weed out the guys who had not committed. This was a huge lesson for me. Go all in, commit, don't be one of the "I'll try-ers," the faint-hearted.

On that Monday when jump school began, we were put into smaller groups, maybe fifty men in a formation. The soldier in front of me and to my left was a West Point graduate who had attained the rank of captain. (In Airborne School there was technically no rank; we were all U.S. Army Airborne volunteers.) I was eighteen years old, and this guy was twenty-four or twenty-five and was sharp and debonair and everything I wanted to grow up to be.

My thoughts went something like this: I could follow this guy into combat any day of the week, and I *will* follow this guy, albeit one step back and one to the right, all the way through Airborne School.

And that's just what happened. He jumped out of the 34-foot tower onto the zip line, and so did I. He went off of the 250-foot tower, and I was next. He went out of the dark rattling airplane, and I was right behind him, drifting to the ground with a big green parachute to keep me from becoming a lawn dart.

They told us in Airborne School that the first jump was always the safest one. Something about how you were concentrating so totally that you had no abstract thoughts interfering, and so you did everything right, by the book. Well, of course not me. And really, I don't think it was my fault. There were two open doors on either side of the airplane, and jumpers were supposed to alternate going out first one and then the other. The jumpmasters—the guys who kick your ass out if you lock up in the doorway—are also the ones regulating the traffic flow.

Okay, so maybe I went through the stop sign just a pinch early, at about the same time a fellow jumper went out the other door. The result was that I ended up going through his lines—the ones connecting him to the parachute canopy—and got tangled in them. Both of our parachutes were inflated so there was no danger. He grabbed my feet and pulled me down to where my feet were at his helmet level. The Army, in its great wisdom, actually trained us for this exact scenario, and there was a sergeant on the ground with a bullhorn, screaming instructions to us both. When we hit the ground, he rolled one way and I rolled the other. And all was right with my world, until they made me do a zillion pushups for being a moron…

Do you remember the exact moment you became self-actualized, when you became a man (if you are one)? The moment you knew you could do anything you put your mind to? In other words, when you discovered you were actually in charge of you.

I do.

And it wasn't jumping out of an airplane.

As our reward for having parachuted five times, they took us for one more run. We were in really good shape by then. So when I tell you it was a real long "we're going to break you" kind of run, you can figure it out.

The drill instructors were running as a relay, so they kept fresh and were able to hold us to a nut-busting pace. After running for a really long time, guys were starting to drop out and throw up, but my eyes were firmly fastened onto my West Point captain's back. The words, "If you can do it, I can do it," kept a steady repeating cadence in my brain.

And then.

He.

My captain.

My hero.

Pulled up, turned out, and puked.

Doing a 180 at 60

Yep, that was the moment I grew up. I've thought of that moment for most of my life, and I guess it was the mental equivalent of having a glass of freezing cold water thrown into my face at the exact moment when my throat was parched and my lungs were burning.

I wondered, "What do I do? Do I follow my captain and quit…or do I keep going?"

I became my own person right then and there and did what I would do every time life became difficult for me. I simply kept putting one foot in front of the other until that particular trial was ended.

I don't know the exact number of parachute jumps I made in the Army, maybe about fifteen. They were all static line jumps, meaning that the parachute is opened by a nylon cord attached to the aircraft with the other end attached to your chute. I jumped out of helicopters, C130s, C119s, and once from a C141 Starlifter jet, which you will see (in a following chapter) has great significance for me.

What a difference I experienced at Eagle Field, located in the San Joaquin Valley in California. It was May 1981, and I was thirty years old as I surveyed the little Cessna 182 I would jump from.

I took a morning ground school, and in the afternoon I did a static line jump from 3,500 feet. (All distances are measured above ground level, not above sea level.) There was no waiting in the door. Oh no. I climbed out the door and hung from the wing strut while being buffeted by the wind, and then I just simply let go.

Two weeks later, I did my first hop and pop, a free fall in which I opened the parachute by myself. Just a quick observation about skydiving: most people think it's about the ride down on the parachute. And although that really is neat, it's not the main focus. It's the short time in freefall (before deploying the chute) that lights up a skydiver's shorts. Why do those moments seem like such a big deal? Perhaps it's because if you don't do something, like pull your own ripcord, you will die in about twenty seconds, no ifs, ands, or buts.

That same year on the Fourth of July, I bombed out of the airplane and was taken off student status to become a certified skydiver. I did my first formation jump along with three others. I did night jumps and many different types of formation jumps, and when I went to open my parachute on jump number sixty-six, it was a malfunction and a bad one. The parachute would not open correctly and was a tangled mess. I had to cut it away at 1,900 feet, which meant pulling a special handle that separated me from the chute and opened my reserve. I touched down on the roof of a house and frantically ran off before my parachute deflated, ending up in someone's backyard. That's how I learned that a reserve chute is not as steerable as a main chute.

In August I did a nude jump from 7,500 feet, along with three others. Damn, I wonder what I was thinking about then. Of course, I wasn't totally nude; I had running shoes on. A year later, I dove out of a Twin Beech at 12,500 feet—my 101st skydive. I had reached my goal of one hundred, and without any sort of advanced planning, I simply stopped skydiving.

I was a pretty accomplished skydiver at thirty-one years old, with something like sixty minutes of actual free fall time. What other sport can you name where you can actually be "accomplished" in about an hour?

* * *

On the morning of August 3, 2011, several months after my 60th birthday, I put on my golfing shoes and went out and played eighteen holes. I slammed down a sandwich and then went out to the garage and fired up my motorcycle. After riding down the mountain and across the valley, I arrived at the Lodi airport and home of the Parachute Center. I went to the counter with my log book in hand and spoke with the owner.

We chatted about my experience, and he remembered many of the guys I used to jump with. He asked what happened to my rig—my parachute and stuff—and I told him I loaned it to a friend many years ago. It was never returned. When I thought about it, I realized that was why I hadn't jumped since: out of sight, out of mind.

The old jumpmaster behind the counter then said something very interesting. "You don't remember what you forgot, but skydiving is so intense that about ten seconds after you start your free fall, it will all come rushing back."

He assigned me to an instructor named Mike who informed me he had about 13,000 jumps under his belt. Holy cow! He ran me through a bunch of positions, mostly proper body arch technique and emergency procedures and such. He also had me practice many times, finding the handle and pulling my pilot chute out. You see, to open your main parachute, you pull out a small pilot chute and release it into the wind. It's attached to the main parachute and when it deploys, it opens your main chute…hopefully. After about two hours of retraining, equipment fitting, and getting dressed, I paid my hundred dollars and followed my instructor to a twin Beech 99 Turboprop airplane.

We quickly climbed to 13,000 feet. While we were climbing to altitude I couldn't help but think about the feeling that a few hours previously I didn't even know if they would let me skydive again after such a long time lapse. Yet here I was, scrunched into another noisy airplane with no door, along with fifteen or so other wild-eyed folks. Mike had a camera mounted to his helmet and shot a video of the entire skydive and landing. He was also there in case I blew it and he had to pull my pilot chute.

Let me state something here most people don't know. There is no feeling of falling when you free-fall. That's because there is nothing relative for you to pass by as you're falling at a rate of about 120 miles per hour. Instead, it appears that the ground is coming up to meet you. Old skydiving joke: it's no big deal when you look down and all of the people look like ants, but you're in deep doo-doo when all of the ants look like people.

The jump was just as the owner promised. It took about ten very intense seconds before it all came flooding back. So perhaps intensity is the key to unlocking long-lost memories, because I was certainly tense, with a pulse rate way up there. I practiced reaching for my ripcord many times on the way down, and after thirty seconds or so we started playing games. I began chasing my instructor around in a circle, left and then right. I kept glancing at my altimeter because you can't help but feel the ground getting closer. At

5,000 feet, I broke off and pulled out my pilot chute, ever so casually tossing it into the wind.

My main parachute opened with a snap. I don't care how many times you do it, there really is a giant sense of relief when you look up and see that colorful canopy above you. That signals the start of the second part of skydiving, namely the parachute ride. I flew my parachute down. That's what you do, because it's really nothing more than a large wing, flown just like a glider. When I reached my target altitude of 1,000 feet, I steered downwind until I was directly above a very busy highway. Then I turned crosswind until I just about reached the hangar, then turned into the wind on final approach. I flared the parachute perfectly and landed on both feet, about as soft a landing as I can remember. Of course, now that the intensity is gone, maybe my memory is back to normal.

There really are no words to describe the feeling when you do something as exciting as skydiving. I never thought of it as cheating death. In fact, I never thought of it as really dangerous, and still don't. If you are in good shape, have good equipment, and train well with a proper attitude, it's a matter of completing something you had already thought through.

It was probably more dangerous riding my motorcycle back home than making the jump itself. I was reminded of that while reliving the jump in my mind and almost missing a corner.

The video of the jump can be viewed on the website JohnRTakacs.com.

* * *

My dad was a true tough-guy paratrooper. On one of his jumps, he cracked his helmet liner when he hit the tail of the airplane, causing permanent hearing loss in one of his ears. He said it was his fault and never went to the VA for treatment.

After retirement he became an alcoholic, something that happens to combat veterans more than you would like to think. He died of kidney failure when he was seventy-eight years old.

Most of him, but not the good part, made it to sixty.

6

Roughing It

On the other side of the street, down the hill and across the field from my boyhood home, was a large wood. When I was younger, I thought it the largest of forests, teeming with wild animals like lions and tigers and bears. Oh my!

It was a giant step in my life when my friend Marty and I pitched a tent in the middle of it (just above a flowing torrent on a huge bluff) and spent the night. Our tent, since we didn't own a real one, was a blanket thrown over a rope tied between two trees. We were not scared, because we were well armed with our BB guns. We were eleven years old.

At that age, we never knew about the philosophical argument of whether a tree makes any noise if it falls in the forest when no one is around. And we sure as hell didn't know that small branches and stuff fall out of the trees all night long and make lots of racket. Really scary racket. We were forever vigilant, no sleep that night.

When I went back to that woods a few years ago, the flowing torrent turned out to be a small brown creek. And the bluff was a hill about fifteen feet high. Of course, there never was any wilder animal than a crazy raccoon or possum.

* * *

When I go for a hike these days, there really are lions (mountain), tigers (panthers), and bears. Now that I think of it, though, the only panther I've seen is Panther Creek Road. Does that mean there once were panthers there?

I would be willing to bet that within a hundred miles of where you live, there is a site/place/thingy that tourists go to visit or see and spend time. And you don't. I was that guy who just kept driving by local attractions until 2005, at age fifty-four. It seems ridiculous to me now that people would come from around the world to enjoy the Sierra Mountains around Lake Tahoe, while just forty minutes away I sat home and let my butt get overly fat. I can't remember exactly why my sweet girl and I decided to change all that, but I'm sure it had to do with spending more quality time together. I think I'll have more to say on "quality" time later.

On our first hike, we set out with Sam, our Golden Retriever, and within ten minutes (or about a half mile), we lost him. Yep, gone. How nice it was of us to let him off the leash. And he reciprocated by chasing after some varmint. We searched for an hour and then headed back to where we parked the car.

There he was, mooching off some other hikers that just thought he was wonderful. He's very cute and I agree he's photogenic...so photogenic that he'll look good in his doggie casket. If something like this has happened to you before (kind of like the time I lost two out of three of my kids at the Smithsonian), you were probably happy to see the missing pet and mad at the same time.

It's times like that, when you look back, that you see what a blessing it was. Because as we continued hiking through the years, we kept Sam on the leash most of the time. One time we were hiking up the back side of Thunder Mountain from Horse Canyon trail. It's about five miles, all uphill—or up-mountain, as it were. We heard a cute meowing coming from a clump of bushes just off the trail. But when you're at

Doing a 180 at 60

10,000 feet elevation and a zillion miles from a house, little kitty cats don't exist. Young mountain lions do. Since Sam was on the leash, we got out of Dodge as fast as our scared butts could manage, before momma mountain lion came back from shopping for food and found it on her doorstep.

Shortly after I turned sixty, my niece and her teen-age children—my grandnieces and grandnephew, otherwise known as my niecettes and nephew-dude—came to visit from Florida. We took them up to the high country and set off on a hike to a small alpine lake.

Not that I'm being judgmental, but most people won't ever see that lake because they've let themselves get too far out of shape. It's not that it's too far for a day hike. It's just that the trail starts at an elevation of almost 8,000 feet. For some, the thin air plus lots of exertion equals a heart attack, too bad. And okay, maybe I am being just a little judgmental.

After we arrived at the lake, we had a mountain snack. Have you ever noticed how everything tastes better when you pack it in? Where else would you take a bite of apple, raw almonds, and cheese and chew it all together and swear it's gourmet food?

After we ate, I climbed up on a rock about twelve feet above the water and did my first back flip of the day into the snow-melt, alpine lake water. I can't remember my first dive off a board, but I would bet it was around the time I took swim lessons. There was a diving board at the Penn High School pool, and I can't help but say it seems that diving boards are a lost source of enjoyment. I haven't seen one in a public pool in many years. I wonder who the no-funner was that decided diving boards are so dangerous that kids aren't allowed to experience them anymore.

All through the years, I've done lots of diving. In grade school and junior high we had ropes hanging from trees over the river, and we would dive off all summer long. In high school, I dove off all the bridges (six, at the time) between County Line Road and Cedar Street in my hometown. The County Line Bridge had old light posts, and we would climb up to the top of the posts and dive off.

I suppose it was technically illegal, kind of like going sixty in a fifty-five zone, which is something most of us seem to do all the time. But really, what was the big deal? We could see up and down the river for a mile. It wasn't as if we were going to dive into somebody's boat or something. And when the sheriff came, what was he going to do? Dive in after us? Or maybe surround the river?

When I enlisted in the Army, my diving exploits continued. I hitched a ride up to a reservoir somewhere

Doing a 180 at 60

in Virginia with my friend and fellow soldier Chuck, and we took a rowboat to some cliffs. Following his lead, I began diving off the rocks at a lower level, working my way up to the top. When I looked down at the rowboat floating innocuously on the water, it seemed about a half inch long. Meanwhile, Chuck, with his lopsided grin, had just dived and was urging me on. I don't know exactly how far it was to the water, maybe eighty or ninety feet, although it looked like five hundred.

I was getting ready to chicken out—cluck, cluck, greasy grimy chicken guts—but while peering over the top, I heard a noise behind me. When I turned around there was a guy in a uniform (forest ranger?), a pretty girl, and another couple there. At the time I really was leaning toward climbing back down. But destiny intruded in the form of the great-looking girl, asking in her cutest-ever southern accent, "Are you really going to dive off here?"

Oh Lord, what a horrible curse, to be thrust into the cute-girl decision-making process. So what would you say? I took the cute-girl bad-decision option.

"Yeah," I answered. And before I could allow another 'fraidy cat thought, I leapt off and went into a graceful swan dive.

Something I had learned through the years was that on the way down you look out at the horizon to keep from flipping over onto your back. Then when you feel the water coming up to meet you, you tuck your head and stick your arms straight over your head and go into your dive.

When I hit the water, I was surprised at how hard it felt, and it pushed my left arm straight down to my side. I was also surprised how shallow my dive was. I thought I would go down fifty feet or so. When I came up, Chuck pulled me into the boat and kept slapping me on the back. He handed me a bottle of Rebel Yell whiskey, only available south of the Mason-Dixon Line. As I took my first hit, he told me I was the only one other than himself who ever dove off the top. You just gotta love paratroopers.

The next day, we began hitchhiking back to the base, and a guy picked us up. He was a complete stranger, but soon enough he and Chuck were drinking buddies, slugging down Rebel Yell whiskey. I was drafted into driving the car, even though I couldn't move my left arm.

With no map I, the Indiana boy, was left to drive alone on unfamiliar roads. Before they both passed out I asked for directions, and all I heard was something about damn Yankees. I finally managed to find my way back to base and drive the stranger's car right up to my barracks. Sometime around four in the morning, I woke them up, got out, and went to bed. What a weekend.

But back to my niecettes and nephew-dude … It's not that kids aren't as adventurous as in days past. They just don't have as many bad examples to follow. So I took care of that. I soon talked them into jumping off the rocks.

You should have seen their little warm-water Florida faces when they came sputtering up from the ice-cold water. Pretty soon they were diving and doing flips off the rocks as if they'd been born to it. I think it was my dad's crazy genes rising to the surface.

Sometimes our hikes are just walks in the forests and mountains, but that day it was more than special. I'm glad I decided to do a 180 with my life so that we could share that moment.

The following morning I had a brilliant idea and called around to find a hole in the ground suitable for crawling about. Ever heard of spelunking? The definition is pretty much in the preceding sentence.

We loaded up and drove over to Murphys, California, ending up at Moaning Cavern. After our safety meeting/pep talk, I harnessed up and rappelled down into the cave, finishing at 165 feet below ground. Of course I'd rappelled before, in the Army. The first time I went off a wall, the second time out of a helicopter, and the third time off a bridge. I really got off on it, and after a while I would go most of the way down without braking until the last few feet.

The cave rappel was different in that it was enclosed, and the special braking mechanism on my harness would only allow me to go slowly, as I pushed the rope through it. However, it was still great fun coming down into the dark main chamber of the cave and landing next to an enormous pile of rubble. We were told the pile was made up of bones of dead humans and animals that had entered the cave without knowing about the huge drop off.

We were outfitted in old jumpsuits (kind of like prisoners wear), knee and elbow pads, and miner's hard hats with lights attached. We crawled down teensy weensy tunnels until we were 275 feet below the earth's surface. I've never been very limber, in fact quite the opposite. With the tight spaces and the tunnel changing direction, I had to be able to turn, sometimes flipping onto my side or back. At first I thought it would be impossible, but once again I was wrong. I should have mentioned we had a guide that showed us how to do it.

Doing a 180 at 60

We came to one part in the cave called the Pancake Squeeze, so named because it was only about a foot tall and four feet wide. I had to get on my back and there wasn't enough room to pull with my arms or push with my legs. That's when I realized we must have been born with an inner snake instinct, because I just kind of slithered through and into the next section called the "birth canal."

There really is a technique to the whole spelunking thing. Beginning on my stomach, I crawled until I came to a rock in the tunnel. There was no way my shoulders would fit through until I twisted sideways and slithered some more. Then I had to turn my shoulders back straight while my hips turned.

There were many unique sections with names like Meat Grinder and Chimney. I'm fortunate that I have never been uncomfortable in tight places, like an MRI tunnel. I've never felt the squeezing sensation that people who are claustrophobic describe. And not once while spelunking did I feel pinched in. But I was concerned—since we were in California—about the question of what would happen in case of an earthquake. Our guide told us that earthquakes are only noticeable at the surface, not deep underground, which made for some relief. It was only later I realized that the only opening to the cave was at the surface...

As for my redo, I spelunked right where I live in the mountains. There are abandoned gold mines, if you know where to look for them. I discovered a few when I was ranging about, and I used to go into them, exploring and looking for gold (as if they would be abandoned with gold lying about). I would take my backpack, loaded with extra batteries and flashlights, tie a strong nylon string to a rock outside, and go into the dark to explore by myself. I know it was dumb, but it was also exciting once the light faded from the tunnel entrance. I never had to get down on my knees and crawl, but when I turned off the light, it was impossible to see my hand in front of my face. I stopped caving alone when I was forty-seven, but I can't seem to remember why. It probably had something to do with a girl.

We finished our spelunking day with a 1,500-foot zip line. A zip line is a cable strung between two towers. After you get into a harness, they attach you to the cable by way of a set of pulleys, and let you go. Gravity does the rest. As I mentioned in the parachute chapter, it was part of our Airborne training, but I hadn't zipped since 1970. For those of you who have never zipped before, I highly recommend it, if for no other reason than to say you've done it. It may also add some exhilaration to your life in a more natural way than a roller coaster could ever compete with.

My niece and her kids went back to Florida at the end of the week, but my sweet girl and I loaded up to go camping and ended up in a large meadow almost at the peak of the Sierras. After a 15-mile hike, we went back to our campsite to rough it.

Sounds exotic, eh? The truth is, we pulled our trailer off the beaten path and had a couple of beers with the pizza we baked in the oven after our hike.

* * *

When Marty and I hung up a couple of old blankets for a tent and slept on the ground, it was just what young kids do. I saw my own kids do it in the living room many times. Simple isn't it? But it seems as I got older I graduated to a motor home, not that I couldn't have pitched a tent. Even at sixty you can redo many things, but you can never duplicate the first-time feeling of adventure that is alive only in a young boy's or girl's heart.

As for my friend Marty, he was a nerd even before the word existed. He went on to graduate from college and always maintained that the only thing he really learned in college was how to party, something he truly needed to learn. I hadn't seen him since high school until October 1987, when I was back in Indiana and had time to go for a walk in our old woods. Can you believe he was home at the same time and we met by accident right in the middle of our woods? Life is pretty cool sometimes.

He made it to sixty.

7

Right on Cue

You may have noticed a lot of sports on my list of things to redo. The designation of "sports" might be a little strong for some of the entries, however. Maybe barroom activities would be a better description. Back in the day, I would spend quite some time playing pool and shuffleboard, horseshoes and pinball.

Even if bowling alleys are not considered bars, you know (if you ever were in a league) that with all the beer frames and such, things seem to turn out the same way. A beer frame, for the uninitiated, is oftentimes the third frame. It can also be any frame when all but one member of your team has a strike in the same frame. The losing member becomes the not-so-lucky buyer.

I really do have a terrific memory, though I can't recall the last time I played pool. But I do remember the first time. Roger, Jerry, and Phil (who were brothers) had a pool table in their basement. For you folks in Cali, a basement is a room (or rooms) under your house. Even though I live in California now, I still can't get used to crawl spaces and slabs.

Playing pool was one reason we were grouped in the basement, but more importantly it was the music and snowy weather. Cold outside, hot inside with the Animals, Beach Boys, Rolling Stones, Beatles, and all of Motown. That's right (on), it was the sixties. It was a time of great discovery. No, not the exploration of the moon, more like shooting moons, driving cars, riding motorcycles, and (wash my mouth out with soap)…girls. I just about died the time Roger's mom yelled as we were heading out to the football game, "You boys keep your peters in your pants." I didn't even know she knew I had one. And as far as pool tables and girls are concerned, well that's a different kind of barroom sport, and it's not going to find its way into this book.

I played lots of pool in my twenties and drank lots of beer. It was during those days I saw the most bizarre thing in my life, and as you know by now, I've seen quite a few. Five of us were killing time at a hippy beer joint in 1976, playing pool and trading dollars around the table. I didn't know any of the guys, but we were just sipping our brews and no one was winning much. We were there for a couple hours, easy. Over in the corner, three girls were drinking (not loud or boisterous or anything), but out of nowhere, one girl got up and walked over to a guy I'd been playing pool with for the past few hours. She started calling him all kinds of foul names and punched him in the face. In pure reaction, he thumped the girl upside the head with the almost empty mug of beer he was holding. She went down and out, as in "thud, out goes the light."

Her two friends came over and dragged her back to their table, and eventually she came to and started drinking again. No one made a big deal out of it, and we continued playing pool. So I asked the guy who was punched what it was all about. He said he'd never seen that girl in his life. It was so surreal, I wondered if there were some type of time glitch and it never really happened.

I had muchos fun playing pool and never saw any real beefs. I think it was the cigarette smoke that finally drove me out of the bars, or it could have been the wife. But really, I *am* allergic to smoke.

* * *

When I was on my coast-to-coast motorcycle trip and was on my way back to California, I stopped in Indiana and met up with some of my old cronies who were scattered about the country, but happened to be home at that time. We got together at the American Legion and decided to play a game of pool, which was slated to be The Most Important Game in the Universe—known and unknown.

Perhaps it is age that keeps us out of the bars or maybe it's our wives. Nope, most of us are single, so it's just got to be our maturity... and fear of a drunk-driving ticket. We were all, at one time, pretty good beer drinkers, and around the table we ordered some lubricating fluid to get us started: Miller Lite, Bud Light, two Coors Lights, and a Diet Coke. After all these years, each of us had sacrificed taste for fewer calories. Now that might make sense if we were pounding down a gallon of the bubbly brew, but come on, two drinks each?

I hadn't played pool in many a year, and getting together with four of my best-est ever friends in the match that would decide the champion of the universe was high pressure. I was trying to concentrate on a difficult straight-in shot while my friends were taking pictures, flashing bright things in my eyes. I was sure they were doing it on purpose, knowing the importance of this particular game.

They were talking and draping their arms around each other the whole time. I mean, it looked like a bunch of old friends who helped each other through the most difficult times of their lives. And they were!

Who would have guessed that the guy you met in the sixth, eighth, or tenth grade would stick to you like glue for the rest of your life? We had been together through marriages, birthdays, kids, jobs, divorces—you name it. But in another sense, was all the talking and back slapping also a psychological ploy to get me to lower my guard? I made that shot, but I was already the winner of the universe, simply by growing older with that bunch of friends.

* * *

Many of our friends were not at that game, and one of them was Jerry's and Roger's youngest brother Phil. When we were growing up, he was the most industrious of us all, with a regular lawn cutting job. Later on, he was highly successful in business, which I have come to understand doesn't mean crap. What? You don't believe me?

Here's a quiz for you, and it only has one correct answer. When Steve Jobs, the great Apple CEO, died at the age of fifty-six, it was estimated his net worth was between ten and twelve billion dollars. How much of that do you think he would give in exchange for life? Correct answer: all of it. Without your health, it will be for naught.

Doing a 180 at 60

My friend Phil died in his early forties of a heart problem.

He never made it to sixty.

8

Rollin' on the River

In writing this, I realized—slowly, of course—how many dumb things I did as a kid, and perhaps even a pinch later. One of those things happened when I was twelve years old. Marty and I had found a half-sunk rowboat in the river that spring. I guess when you're a kid, you think a half-sunk abandoned boat belongs to those who recover it. I'm pretty sure I read in some now-banned Huck Finn book about international salvage rights or something.

How the two of us scrawny kids dragged it out of the water and carried it inland over a half mile, I sure as heck can't recall. But we did. It probably had something to do with the old adage, "Where there's a will, there's a way." We hid the boat under a big tree and covered it with brush until we gathered up some paint. Then we painted the boat and built some home-made oars. But after we had put in all that work—and just before our great debut—some pirates came along and swiped our swiped boat.

You would think that would serve as a warning to me about things that float on the water. But no.

Years later I bought a house on the river, and my friend Aaron brought his canoe over for storage. I kept it upside down in my yard so it wouldn't fill up with rainwater. One evening Aaron and my brother came over with some beer in a cooler, and we headed downstream in the canoe. We ended up in a little creek where eventually we ran out of water, meaning the creek was dried up. So we turned around and headed back to deep water.

Somehow water started coming into the canoe. Lo and behold, ants had built a nest in the upside-down canoe, and they came boiling out by the zillions. We all bailed out into the river and had to tread water until we capsized the canoe and drowned all the ants. Even so, while we were in the water, we became ant islands with those creatures crawling on our heads and faces. The thought of it still creeps me out.

Later on another friend (Bobby) and I decided we wanted to be in the big canoe race from South Bend, Indiana, to Niles, Michigan. I was working construction at the time and was probably in the greatest physical shape of my life. Bobby was also in great shape, with big strong arms. One small—and I thought, insignificant—problem was that he had never canoed before. And you just read the sum total of my canoeing experience.

Since I was the more experienced, I sat in the back as the steersman. The race started and off we went like a shot out of a poorly aimed gun. We zoomed straight across the river and ran into the other bank. Really, I thought, how hard can this be? We set off again, bridge dead ahead, but it had a forty to fifty foot space to get our skinny little boat through. No matter how I tried to steer, though, I was going to hit the freaking bridge.

I yelled, "Stop paddling!"

With only inches to spare, we missed the huge concrete abutment. By then we were in last place and we both started to get the paddling thing down. This helped us start catching up to the other canoes. However, I couldn't help but notice the other guys were only paddling one smooth stroke to our three or four… or ten.

And then we started across the river again and barely stopped before hitting the other bank. We were sweating like great Viking sailors trying furiously to catch the little old ladies up ahead, who looked like they were bird watching or something. When we finally crossed the finish line, I knew we won. Because no matter what they say, we paddled at least twice as far as anybody else. We figured for sure someone bribed the judges, when we found out we took last place in our division.

I also went canoeing up in Northern Michigan one time in 1994 with my brother-in-law Ray and some younger guys. It was a kick-ass time, with lots of beer drinking. For some reason, I was not allowed to steer. So when earlier this summer my sweet girl and I went canoeing on a cold water lake up here in the mountains, that redo sums up my entire canoeing experience. I'm proud to say I survived.

And then there is kayaking, which was truly on my written goal list for twenty years. I did it for the first time in 2004 on the ocean at Catalina Island and again recently.

But my best rowing experience (can you guess?) was white-water rafting. The first time I went rafting was in the early spring on the Yuba River in Northern California. I was thirty-four (1985) and had only been living in California for a few years. I had no clue where we were going. The surprise probably showed in my eyes when we got there and they made us put on wet suits. The river guide calmly told us how people get killed doing this kind of thing. He also explained that when you see all the white water, it's really just air churned up in the water, the same air that won't allow your life jacket to float you to the top if you go under.

I began thinking about my entire row-row-row-your-boat experience up to that point, which was to say, calm water. There is really no comparison between that and truly exciting white-water rafting. It's not even close.

White-water rafting is like being bipolar. One moment you're in a great calm stretch of water, and the next moment you're hurtling through rapids. I only remember one of the serious spots in the river, aptly named the Maytag. The name alone should give you an idea of what it was like. With our experienced guide we went churning through, and it was an adrenaline fueled feat. After awhile, we knew when we were coming to a bad spot in the river, because of all the people sitting on the rocks on the riverbank watching like looky-loos at an accident scene. I went rafting many times after that and always had a great time, but once again stopped as I got older. I don't know why, but sure wish I did.

* * *

My niece and niecettes came visiting from Florida a year after their first visit. In my goal to complete the process of corrupting them, I talked them into going skydiving. Instead of hating it, they became addicts.

The following day, I called and made a white-water rafting reservation for the south fork of the American River. This was a summertime white-water trip, when the river typically is not so wild, and the sun is good and hot.

This would be an easy trip—no wet suits and just floating freely down the river, finishing at Folsom Lake. At this time, however, it might be a good idea to reread the third paragraph of this chapter.

It had been a terrific day and we were getting close to the end, with one last technical section to go. It was called the Hospital Zone or something like that. I was in the front of the raft when we went over a ten-foot waterfall, plunged straight down, and crashed into a giant hydraulic jump wave at the bottom. Hooked into the raft only by sliding my right foot under a strap, I was pitched into the wild, foaming, angry, churning river for the first time in my rafting career. I hit my elbow on a rock and came up pointing feet first down the rapids, just the way our guides had instructed.

Aye, me mates started rowing the boat back toward me, and I climbed back in, laughing my head off. The guide told us later that our raft folded like an accordion in the middle.

* * *

My mom has always said she had three families with one husband. My three sisters were much older than my brother and me, and my younger sisters came much later. My older brothers-in-law were present in my oldest memories, since they started hanging around my sisters when I was six or seven years old. Because they had always been around, I always thought of them as my brothers.

Ray was my oldest brother-in-law and was a super good guy. He served in the Navy and was actually stationed in Cuba during the Cuban Missile Crisis. He was a great example of following the American dream, starting as a carpenter and progressing to a building contractor and successful business owner.

Ray was only fifty-eight years old when he had a heart attack and died, just two weeks after a physical examination pronounced him fit and healthy.

He never made it to sixty.

9

Swim, Bike, Run. Repeat

You know about my swimming. And my first bike ride may still be fresh in your mind. What about running?

Red Ball Jets: run faster, jump higher. Does anybody remember that commercial? Red Ball sneakers were called tennis shoes back then, what we now call running shoes. Maybe it was a local commercial, and I remember the shoes because my mom worked at Ball Band Corporation where they were made. When Mom brought me home a pair, I strapped those babies on and was off like a jet.

I was a little disappointed after running around and tripping over a fallen tree I had tried to jump over. I suppose my jet motor quit working or something. I was okay, barely bleeding, and everybody thought I was so cute telling my sad story. I think we should have sued the bastards for malpractice, malfeasance, or malnutrition. Wait a minute, I keep forgetting: that was back when we took responsibility for our own actions.

Anyway, swim, bike, run: triathlon.

So when was my first triathlon? Follow me on this one. Even though the first official triathlon event was in San Diego in 1974, when do you think I participated in my first triathlon? Remember, I grew up on a golf course with a river running through it. It was a municipal course, which means the city owned it. So it wasn't exactly *legal* to be on the golf course. But here's a small technicality. They didn't own the river, just the land bordering it.

The city employed a park cop who drove around in a little, orange, three-wheeled Cushman scooter. When we saw him, we would swim to the bank and scramble out of the river, run as fast as we could across the golf course, jump on our bikes, and race off with the cop in hot pursuit. So you see, we actually invented the triathlon in the 1950s. The prize was not a medal or trophy but consisted of avoiding some serious hard time in a dank dark jail cell, to be sure. My dad told me so.

When I came back from Vietnam with a badly broken foot in 1971, my therapy was to swim. So the Army, in its great wisdom, made me a lifeguard. Since this was my job, I had to arrive early at the lake and swim with the other lifeguards as part of our PT (physical training). My longest nonstop swim was a mile. During that wild summer—it was the year I dove off the cliff—I actually saved three people from drowning. Remember, though, it was my job, and I had been trained and certified to do so.

* * *

I had not swum any appreciable laps since that time forty years before, when I decided to sign up for my first official triathlon. (If it sounds strenuous, difficult, and dumb, sign me up.) In 2011, I had spent the summer doing lots of biking and running, so I thought, "What's the big deal about swimming some laps, huh?"

I swam the twenty-five yards to the end of the pool and then swam back. And just about died. I couldn't get over how hard it was, but decided to continue training anyway. After that first training day, I increased my distance a few laps every other day. When I got to twenty laps (five hundred yards), I would rest. Then I started adding more laps and sets.

Within three weeks I swam my first nonstop mile. Now to be sure, I would do as many freestyle laps as I could and then go to breaststroke to rest, then back to freestyle. However, now I can swim a mile nonstop using only freestyle. In fact, I took a class to learn how to swim in the Total Immersion way.

Total Immersion swimming is about getting long and lean, swimming on top of the water with less drag. Also it specifies just one kick per stroke, which keeps you from wearing your legs out, a great advantage in a triathlon. Of course, there's much more to it than that, and you can research it online for more information. With Total Immersion, I have increased my stamina to swim more than two and a half nonstop miles.

Since I now had my swimming down, I thought it would be a good idea to do a longer run before I entered my first triathlon. So my sweet girl and I decided to enter a 10K race. She ran once in a while, but had never run in a real race. To hear her talk, she's not very competitive... She went online and started following a very structured plan to train for the 10K. Walk a little, run a little, and slowly increase the amount of time spent running, just like the Army taught. Please, what did she know?

Instead, I went out and ran four miles and pulled my hamstring muscle. She kept building up; I kept sitting in the chair, resting with ice, compression, elevation. Hey, RICE is an acronym for resting, ice, compression, elevation. Maybe I invented something. I got over the pulled muscle slowly.

After a lifetime of strenuous activity, I have tweaked, torn, twisted, and strained just about every muscle in my body. I'm not sure it takes any longer to heal now than it used to. They all eventually heal, because even after the age of sixty, we heal.

We did our 10K in Big Sur, and I finished limping. She smoked me. No big deal, because six weeks later we entered a half marathon, 13.1 miles, another redo. I had run one other half marathon when I was thirty-one years old. I don't remember my time, but I did run it with my friend Davey. I was five or six years older than he was, and he used to call me Old Man when we were into something difficult and I was struggling. It's ironic that I was called Old Man at thirty-one, and now I was almost twice that age and running a half marathon again.

Since it was unseasonably cold (twenty-eight degrees at start time), I had on my gloves, stocking cap, and jacket. I watched my sweet girl's cute butt disappear ahead of me into the crowd, and then I started running. After two miles, I unzipped my jacket. My gloves came off a short time later. And then I took off the jacket and tied it around my waist.

I was somewhere around the seven mile mark, going up a big hill, when I saw Davey running next to me out of the corner of my eye.

Doing a 180 at 60

He said, "Come on, Old Man, let's go."

I said out loud back to him, "Okay, let's go."

The girl in front of me turned around and looked at me strangely.

I wasn't hallucinating and I'm not crazy. I'm telling you: he was there. Even though he had died years before, I could feel his presence. I know about runner's high, and I can even give myself a squirt of adrenaline on demand, but this was different. I increased my pace and Davey ran with me. After one more "Come on, Old Man," he disappeared, just before the finish line. That was when my sweet girl, tired of waiting for me at the finish line, ran back to meet me. (Not competitive, my ass.) After I finished, I sat down on the curb with tears in my eyes.

I have a picture of me after my first half marathon thirty years ago, sitting on a curb with my head in my hands. I don't think there was any difference in how beat I felt then as compared to now.

In case you're wondering, my sweet girl beat me by twenty-five minutes in her very first half marathon. I would have made her walk home except that she drove.

Lucky me.

* * *

My first official triathlon was sponsored by our health club and was called "Just TRI." They labeled it as a mini-triathlon, and it was composed of a ten-mile exercise bike ride, a three-mile run around the parking lot, and a thirty-lap swim in the pool. I couldn't believe how strangely difficult it was. But it was the start, for me, of a fascinating new love affair.

Up next was an Olympic distance triathlon. In Europe it's called a 5150, which is the total distance in the metric system. If you go to an emergency room in California and get labeled a 5150, you are a crazy person. Yep, sounds about right to me.

With twelve days to go before the triathlon, and on a Sunday morning while running up a steep hill, I twanged my left hamstring muscle again, without any warning. I treated it with lots of RICE: rest, ice, compression, and elevation. Easy does it. The next day I went to the pool and swam 300 yards as a warm-up and then 1,400 yards freestyle. But this was weird, because my time was only one minute slower. How could my leg hurt so badly that I could barely walk, yet I could still swim almost as fast as before the injury? I know there are different muscles involved, but aren't your legs still your legs?

I guess this is as good a place as any for this statement: I think as you get older, running is the hardest of all the sports. I believe it's the impact that makes it so. Funny, but I had a podiatrist who told me, "Every time you run, it does permanent damage to your feet."

I looked at the short, overly fat doctor and said, "I think being overweight is much worse. If you die of a heart attack from just sitting around, it doesn't matter what your feet are like."

A few days after my running injury, my hamstring felt worse, and I started to get really worried. I first tore my left hamstring at the age of thirty-six while dirt-bike riding, and since that time I've had trouble with tightening. I spent two days researching muscle strains and learning everything I could about them.

What I came up with was Active Release Technique. It's what many Ironman triathletes do for bad soft-tissue injuries. I found a doctor about sixty miles away and began therapy, which involves breaking up scar tissue inside the muscle. After my first Active Release Technique treatment I felt better. Two days later I had a second treatment, and most of my pain was gone.

While recovering, I stopped running and started using an elliptical machine instead. After one bike ride in the rolling hills, I also gave up on the real bicycle and stuck to easy pedaling on the exercise bike with high RPMs—spinning, in the bike world. By this time, I didn't care about my performance during the triathlon. I just wanted to be able to finish safely. I did keep swimming, as I couldn't feel much pain, although my kick felt weak.

Finally, the big day arrived: Sunday morning, Race Day. I prepared all of my racing gear and ate my normal breakfast, a smoothie. It contains tons of protein, good fat, and lots of carbs. We got to the race an hour early, and after checking in I set up my transition area on a towel next to a fence and nervously awaited the start.

First would be the swim, which I was most confident about. We all got in the water for a brief warm-up swim, and then it was 10…9…8, yeah, yeah GO. All amped up, I began swimming. Twenty yards out, I got kicked in the jaw. It felt like the worst punch I'd ever taken, but I knew it wasn't on purpose. A small snort of water up the nose and I came around and somehow got into the breaststroke while I waited for the departure of the Milky Way. I tried to begin my overhand swim stroke, but had trouble getting air, so I continued the breaststroke for about two hundred yards. As I started to feel better, it didn't help to see all of the swimmers in a pack, way ahead of me.

My overall triathlon goal was to finish, but not in last place. Pretty simple. After seeing the swimmers traveling in a pack ahead of me, I was afraid to look behind and see if I was last. I got into my rhythm and was going pretty well when the gal in the kayak pulled up beside me and told me I was off course. I was swimming into the sun and had lost sight of the buoy. I made a small course correction and only added a couple hundred yards to my 1,600 yard swim (making my distance almost a mile, which is 1,760 yards). As I made my turn around the buoy that was the two-thirds marker, I looked back and there were other swimmers behind me. Somehow that pumped me and I began to swim faster.

I finished the swim and came out of the water to run up the hill to the start of the biking portion, but my "run was only a walk. My run legs were out to lunch.

When training for the triathlon, I was swimming in a pool and averaging about two minutes for 100 yards and calculated it would take thirty-three minutes for the swim. I had figured I might get off course and told my sweet girl it would probably be thirty-five minutes. My time was actually 35:43. That makes me wonder about setting expectations. Next time, I think I'll aim for thirty minutes.

When I reached the transition area, I had to put on my jersey, socks, bike shoes, helmet, and sunglasses.

I'd been practicing for a few days and did everything just the way I was supposed to—a good omen.

Generally, I like the bike ride best, but was worried about not having ridden for the previous few weeks. It only took a couple of miles before I could feel the long layoff in my legs as I was going up a big, long hill. Then my bike started to skip out of gear. It started up-shifting in the hardest part of the hill, making it much more difficult to pedal. There I was, out in the middle of nowhere, cussing up a storm. In addition, the temperature started getting really hot. (After we left the race, the thermometer in the car showed ninety-nine degrees.)

I hung in there and even enjoyed a bit of it now and then, mostly when I was coasting down hills. I finished the 24.6 mile bike ride in an hour and thirty-eight minutes. My fastest practice time on the same course was an hour and twenty-eight minutes. Of course, that was without swimming nearly a mile beforehand.

Once again, I was in the transition area where I changed my shoes, took off my helmet, put on a hat, and snapped on a belt that had my race number attached. I had a strategy for the run: walk the uphills, jog the steep downhills, and run the flats. Even practicing, I had never gone this far, and after a half mile

Doing a 180 at 60

I thought my left calf muscle would explode. It was as tight as I had ever experienced in my entire life.

At the water station, the attendant suggested some electrolyte, which she mixed up and gave me. The attendant happened to be Laurie, my triathlon mentor. She saved me. Within minutes the cramp went away and I could actually run the flats and downhills, although when trying to run uphill my hamstring would start yelping. At the five-and-a-half mile mark, my hamstring had had enough and started to unwind. I slowed to a walk, and after a few minutes of babying it, the spasm released. The finish was downhill and I ran to the finish line, double-dang proud of myself.

Speaking of dang, a short time later while loading my bicycle onto the carrying rack of the car, the bicycle's back wheel fell off. Apparently some dang guy who replaced the rear tire a few days before had forgotten to tighten the axle properly. Luckily, that same dang guy didn't crash out there on the course. Maybe double-dang lucky!

When I first began training for the triathlon, I wanted to run the 6.2 miles in about an hour. After I hurt myself, I realistically thought I could make it in an hour and forty-five minutes or (please, dear God) maybe an hour and a half. It was a real shock when I completed the run in one hour and fourteen minutes.

Even more shocking, they called my name for first place in the men's over-sixty age bracket. I guess when there is no one else over sixty in your class, it's automatic. As I thought about it, I came to realize I was not only the sole entrant in my class, but also the oldest racer that day. I think that says a lot, don't you?

So where did I go from there? Sure, I did some more Olympic distance triathlons, but what about the pinnacle of all competitions, the Ironman?

You know how things seem to start so innocently. My friend Laurie and I were riding our bicycles one sunny fall day and out of nowhere I said, "Hey, we should do a half Ironman next year." (Ironman is a Registered Trademark.)

She was quiet a moment and then said, "Okay, but it has to be early in the year, before summer."

You see? So simple. Remember those words.

Simple, sure. But not easy. The next six months of almost full-time training for the half Ironman was about as difficult as learning rocket science. I think it's because you have three totally different sports to fit into one space-time continuum. The reality of it all is you never feel like you're putting enough time into any of the disciplines.

We signed up for the 2013 Ironman 70.3 Boise, Idaho. The half Ironman, called the Ironman 70.3, consists of a 1.2-mile swim, 56-mile bike and a half-marathon run of 13.1 miles. Add it all together and it comes 70.3 miles.

After my last swim start, I thought well… maybe bad luck. The swim start in an Ironman is physically brutal, although not intentionally so. It's just that you have hundreds of swimmers taking off from the same place, and there are no lines on the bottom of the lake to guide you to stay in your lane, as there would be in a swimming pool. Swimmers swim over you, under you, and into you. And they kick you. And you do the very same thing. At first it made me angry, but eventually for some odd reason it started to crack me up. I could feel a smile starting, even underwater. I guess it could be the residual effect from that kick in the jaw in my first triathlon.

When we came out of the water, we lay down on a carpet and the Ironman crew stripped our wetsuits off in one clean jerk. That was a good thing, since I have a hard time getting out of mine. (If the water temperature is 76.1 degrees Fahrenheit or colder, wetsuits are allowed. And this Ironman was one of them.)

The bike portion was a bit windy and somewhat hilly, and the only thing I did wrong was forget to stop at the last aid station for water. I totally ran out with seven or eight miles to go. I can't describe the feeling of reaching down for a water bottle I thought was full and instead finding it empty.

Having no water cramped me up, and I didn't even realize it until I got off the bike and prepared for the run. I took one step and my legs went into a cringing spasm. It was the worst pain I ever experienced, and all I could think about was: one step down, thirteen miles minus one step to go.

I started chugging water and salt pills. For the first mile, I would jog fifty feet and then stop to un-cramp. It kept getting better each mile (not to say it wasn't still extremely painful) and somehow I managed to hang on and finish. It was definitely one step in front of the other. Even after I finished, I was pretty angry at myself for forgetting the water. I felt like I had wasted the last six months of hard training.

So when Laurie called me several months later and said, "We need to do the 2015 Boulder, Colorado Ironman next summer," I was all in. You see? Time heals all.

I told you it always starts out simple.

Then she called in January and said, "If we sign up now, we can get into the 2015 Santa Cruz, California Ironman (otherwise known as the Big Kahuna) next fall." Hey, I'm all in.

Doing a 180 at 60

So here's what happened. I decided to drive to Boulder for the Ironman, which I did and finished. I told my friend Aaron about it and he said, "Hey, the following weekend I'll be in Bowling Green, Kentucky, for a big drag race." At sixty-seven years old, he still drag races a '55 Chevy. Afterward he was going to his brother's house in Indiana. I thought that since we were getting older, it would be good to spend some time with him. We all know how it can happen so quickly and, sure enough, one week after we said goodbye, Aaron had a heart attack and ended up with a triple bypass and a pig valve.

So simple.

I was worried about falling out of shape by being away so long, and after looking at the Ironman website, I couldn't help but notice a race in Muncie, Indiana, just a few (or maybe a hundred) miles from where I was going to be. It was only a week after I said goodbye to my friend, so I signed up and finished that one. Boulder on June 13, Muncie on July 11, and Santa Cruz coming up on September 13. I needed something in August.

So simple.

Ironman Lake Stevens, Washington, just popped up on the map for August 16.

I finished four Ironman 70.3 competitions within three calendar months and figured I set a new world record for an over sixty-year-old. Maybe it's not an official world record, but in the world we now live in, if I say it's so, then it is.

Actually, according to Ironman, I'm the first sixty-four-year-old to do such, and the second guy in his sixties to have done so.

I have gone on to complete nine Ironman 70.3 triathlons and even qualified for the world championships that took place in Australia. I am still in complete amazement that in five years I went from way out of shape to an All World Athlete, an Ironman designation.

* * *

My close friend Sam (Aaron's younger brother) was one of the original golf course triathlon inventors, always looking around for golf balls and running from the "heat." When I was eight years old, he saved me from drowning after I stepped on a floating pallet I thought was a dock.

Sam served with the Marine Corps in Vietnam. He came home a little troubled and graduated to become a skid row drunk. He disappeared for years, but eventually (with God's help, his words) pulled out of his death spiral and became sober.

Doing a 180 at 60

As he grew older, he would still throw golf clubs—which would sail like small helicopters—whenever he hit a lousy shot.

Sam died of terminal liver cancer. He truly found peace in his life and made it to the age of sixty-two.

He did make it to sixty. The problem was he didn't remember half of it.

10

Food, Glorious Food

This seems a good time to talk about food, as promised.

I should have some kind of disclaimer here so you guys don't sue my butt off. How's this? I'm not trying to change anyone's diet or way of eating. This is just some of the stuff I've learned over the years, much of it the hard way. And it worked for me.

Many people promote their view of food as gospel truth. They think (or perhaps feel) that their view is holy and right. Not me. Each and every one of us is different.

When I first started my Seven Cs diet, it was really just to cut down on sugar in my diet, not cut it completely out of my diet. In 2011 my weight dropped from its high point of 225 pounds down to 185 pounds with the Seven Cs diet. To put that in perspective,

Doing a 180 at 60

when I got out of the Army in 1972, I weighed 177 pounds. Essentially, I gained fifty pounds in forty years, most of it after I turned fifty.

That first year after my forty pound loss in 2011, I gained back twelve pounds when winter came, in spite of continuing to work out often—just not as much as before.

The next year I decided to drop all the "whites" and fat from my diet. My weight that summer actually increased a bit to 200, before it dropped to a low of 196.

That following winter, I went up to 212 pounds. I couldn't believe it. I was still working out. So that year I decided to go back to my Seven Cs diet, and I dropped back to 196. Are you seeing a pattern here?

Every summer I lost weight, but not as much as before. And every winter I gained. I really wanted to believe I was gaining muscle, but I went to the tank for the underwater weighing fat test, and it wasn't so.

I have been studying diet now for many years. I understand the linear scale that places vegans on one end of the scale and Paleos on the other, with the vegetarians just inside the vegan territory and the LCHF (Low Carb High Fat) folks just inside the Paleos. Most of us are somewhere in the middle.

But what's the truth? Is it simply that I was fat and lazy with no will power?

Well, you know from reading this I'm not lazy, and to keep doing what I'm doing takes tremendous will-power. So why was I still overly fat? The next winter (2014) when my weight hit 217 pounds, I was ready to try anything that didn't involve surgery or death.

I read *The Big Fat Surprise* by Nina Teicholtz. And then *Good Calories, Bad Calories* by Gary Taubes. Then I read *The Art and Science of Low Carbohydrate Living* by Dr. Stephen Phinney and Dr. Jeff Volek and many more, which was how I became a Low Carb High Fat convert.

Essentially I gave up all sugar, no big deal since I pretty much did that on my Seven Cs diet. But it was a big deal to give up the grains: wheat, rice, corn, and oats. I also rid myself of simple starches, mostly from potatoes and such.

So what was the result? In no real hurry my weight dropped down to 184, but the remarkable thing was that I wasn't crazy hungry anymore. Checking in with the tank, I discovered it was thirty-three pounds of fat that came off.

My official numbers for blood pressure, HDL, and triglycerides are astonishingly good. I take my pulse first thing every morning with a heart rate watch.

Doing a 180 at 60

My normal pulse has fallen to around 45 beats per minute. The reason I take my pulse first thing is that when it gets to the mid-fifties, I know I am tired or over trained. That's when I need to back off for a day or two.

Here's the bottom line, though: I feel good. The arthritis in my wrist, knees, and other places has totally disappeared.

Is it the diet or the exercise? Probably both. And does it really matter as long as it's gone?

If you are overly fat and want to do something about it, talk to your physician, do some research, and decide if it's time for you to do a 180.

11

Who's Your Caddy?

You probably saw this chapter coming. After all, growing up on the golf course and not playing golf would be like growing up in a monastery and not...eating. It seems the mental picture I have of monks is that they were all overly fat. Come to think of it what did those monks eat? Perhaps they should have read my previous chapter.

In 1960, when I was nine years old, I showed up at the golf course clubhouse all by myself and rented a set of golf clubs. Since I had no clue what I was doing, I was paired with a really, really old man and woman. They were probably about sixty years old at the time. They were very kind to me and helped me select which club to use, since I didn't know the difference between a three iron and a putter. (Many years later, that kindness would be repaid in a most unexpected way.)

Back in those days, my buddies and I played in the morning before nine o'clock for fifty cents each. If the club's goal was to create an addiction that would last a lifetime, they succeeded, and much can be learned from that example of how to create and keep customers.

I can remember when my goal was to beat 180 strokes on the score card, trying to take fewer than ten swings per hole. Then the goal was whittled down to 125 strokes for eighteen holes of golf. It was a major deal when I hit 100, and each time thereafter that I lowered my score by another ten strokes—down to the 90s, 80s, and finally the 70s. I would go to the golf course every day and look for balls in those days. And in the evenings, my buddies and I would take one club and practice. Every so often we would sneak in a round of speed golf.

What, you never heard of speed golf? Here's how we played. We would start late, when it was almost dark. Only one club (usually a five iron) and two balls were allowed. On the first tee, we would hit our balls simultaneously—ready, set, go—and then run after them. Hit 'em again and keep going, watching out behind for our buddies' balls to come flying or rolling past. We had to putt, chip, and drive with our one and only beat-up secondhand club. If we lost a ball we could use our spare, but if we lost that one, any ball we could find would come into play.

You had to have a strategy, because there were some holes where you could always find a ball and some where you couldn't. The holes that crossed the river were deadly. The winner was the person who finished first with the lowest number of strokes, although I think it was more important to finish first than to have the fewest strokes. It only took about an hour to play eighteen holes and we would finish sweaty. Many times we would get tackled while running down the fairways. It was great fun.

Remember a few paragraphs ago when I spoke of repayment? It was a hot summer day in my twenty-seventh year (1978). I wanted to get a round in, but I was painting the trim on my house and was about to give up on playing, having worked through prime time so to speak. I finally finished and, not knowing why, headed to the golf course. I hadn't played that late since I was a kid. It was after five o'clock when I started my round of golf. I was by myself, just beating balls and playing two to three balls per hole on the mostly deserted golf course I grew up on.

Doing a 180 at 60

I noticed an elderly couple behind me, walking and pulling hand carts. When they started to catch up, I would play a little faster. On the back nine, I took my shoes off and meandered into the creek, looking for balls, and then sped up again when I saw the older folks closing in on me.

I was on the 16th green practicing my putting when I heard some yelling. I tried to put it out of my serious golf-putting mind, thinking it was just some kids hollering. I finally looked backward and understood that what I was hearing was the word "help." Other golfers were running toward the 15th green and from where I stood could not see. I don't know how I knew, but I instantly took off running. When I came across the top of the hill separating the 15th green from the 16th tee, I could see the old man flat on his back.

I ran the 350 yards separating us and wasn't out of breath at all. The old man's face was turning purple, but I recognized him as the older man who had helped me learn to play golf all those years ago. I asked the two people who were standing over him if they gave him any mouth-to-mouth or CPR. They said they didn't know how.

Thank you, Army, for getting me wounded, making me a lifeguard, and teaching me how to save a life. I went to work on the guy and got him breathing, but then he stopped again. Pretty soon a woman came to help and with the two of us doing the chest reps and the mouth-to-mouth, we brought him back.

Finally the ambulance came and carted him off to the hospital. I ended up taking his and his wife's pull-behind golf carts home with me. It must have been quite a sight, seeing me cross the golf course pulling three carts hooked together like a choo-choo train.

I received "you done good, boy" letters from the mayor and police chief for my good deed. But the coolest thing was that the old man recovered. For many years I got a fruit basket from Florida and a card, thanking me and saying if it wasn't for me... well, you know.

So what did my friends say?

"Hey, we hear you like kissing old men."

I swear, sometimes I think life would be so much simpler if you had no friends, but a lot less exciting.

* * *

When it came time to figure out my golf redo, saving a life on the course was a pretty hard act to follow. And since I lived across the street from another golf course and played all the time, I wondered what I could redo. That's when I remembered that during one summer in my early teens, my goal was to play 100 rounds of golf. I don't think I ever accomplished that. If I had, I wouldn't have forgotten, since I would have bragged about it to my friends. So in my sixtieth year I decided to play 100 rounds of golf.

At sixty, you're supposed to be past your best golf days. I don't know if it's the new technology or what, but I seem to be hitting the ball farther than ever. In my twenties, I became pretty strong and developed a slice, mostly because I couldn't swing the club inside out anymore. Well, that cured itself, and I have a nice little draw most of the time.

I played my lowest round ever this year (76 on a par 72), and separately my two lowest nine-hole rounds (38 on a 37 par on the front nine and an even par of 36 on the back). I actually had lower scores before, but I didn't totally know the rules of golf like I do now. In other words, I was an unintentional cheater.

I have been hit many times by golf balls, but two times come to mind as noteworthy. Once was when I was behind a big boulder and thought I could hit over it. I hit a hard five iron and the ball hit the rock and came back and hit me in the chest. It hurt like hell and left a big red welt. That ball dropped almost straight down and I had to hit it again. I chose a wedge the next time, and my friend told me I had my eyes closed when I swung at the ball and missed it by a foot.

The other notable injury happened after I hit a killer drive and was walking up the cart path. On the previous hole, the tee was over a small hill and a ball came out of nowhere, hit the cart path directly in front of me, and then bounced up, striking me right square in the you-know-where. In a higher octave voice, I yelped, but continued and four-putted that hole, and kind of lost my mojo.

But back to my goal in 2011: I made it. I had more than a hundred rounds that year for the first and only time ever. The volume definitely helped my game, especially putting, but the greatest part of it was spending all that time with my cronies. And lying about how great a golfer I could have been, if'n only.

* * *

My golfing friend Bryon was my rival in our younger years. He lived on an adjacent street and when our gang (armed with crab apples) went to start a big gang fight, his gang was ready to poke sticks in our bicycle wheels. I'm not sure what would have happened next. Probably apple sauce. Luckily they chickened out, something I remind him of quite often.

We were probably enemies because he went to a private school and also I never saw him get spanked like the rest of us. For some reason, when we were spanked together it always made us better friends, like blood-butt brothers or something. He and I got together in high school and became lifelong friends. In high school, Bryon was lousy golfer—and worse, a club thrower—but he was a really good football player.

However, it was his younger brother Kevin who was the real thing: big and fast, a real talent. Life is so weird sometimes and unfair, because when Kevin was in high school he had a stroke. Like most stroke victims, his left arm and leg didn't work correctly anymore. But the worst part was that it erased his memory, and he had to learn everything all over again. He went on to recover somewhat, get married, and live a productive life until suddenly his heart gave out. He died in his fifties.

He never made it to sixty.

12

The Wild Blue Yonder

Yonder, according to the dictionary, means something that is a more or less distant place. As you will read, it describes my experience exactly.

It isn't there anymore, but growing up we had a small airport a couple of miles from where we lived. My friend Ross and I showed up one day and chartered our own plane and pilot. That's the real truth. We were in the seventh grade and it was 1964. I was thirteen years old.

We were nosing around, looking at the airplanes, when one of the pilots showed up and we asked him to take us for a ride. He asked if we had any money, and between the two of us we had six dollars. Once again, no parental consent, just cold hard cash, and we were soon soaring off the ground. My life would never be the same.

Doing a 180 at 60

I still remember that day when we flew around our own little world, which suddenly became much larger and at the same time much smaller. Larger because I was sure I could see all the way to Florida where we had just been vacationing a few weeks before. Smaller because we were looking down when we flew over my house, and the golf course wasn't *way* across a huge field. It was just across a small open area. We flew over the Golden Dome at Notre Dame University, and it seemed like the gold was liquid and flowing down it. I couldn't believe the river had so many twists and turns. Swimming in it all the time, I only knew of one turn.

I was thrilled when we landed because I knew that my flying days had just begun. It's strange to look back and realize that flight also ignited my passion for reading. I began reading everything I could lay my hands on that had to do with flying. In all honesty, reading is also what caused me to become a writer. What an amazing rate of return for a six-dollar investment.

* * *

It was Valentine's Day 1971, and at nearly twenty years old, I was once again flying. But now it was for my country. I was a crew chief/gunner on a UH-1 (Huey) helicopter. When the recruiter signed me up for the Army, I thought I signed up to be a pilot. Oops, someone fibbed. It didn't really matter, because I got some front-seat time and learned how to fly enough to save my life. I was planning to apply for flight school once I returned from Vietnam.

On that fateful day, my company (a part of the 158th aviation battalion, 101st Airborne Division) was directly in the middle of a large battle. The operation was called Lam Son 719, and we were resupplying the South Vietnamese army in Laos. That day we flew out of Khe San, our temporary forward base. It was the same base the marines fought a terrible battle for in 1968. Inside, the helicopter was stacked from the floor to the roof with small arms ammunition, machine gun bullets, grenades, and other things that go boom.

We landed on a small hill inside the border of Laos, and I had just kicked back, stretching my legs out in front of me on an ammo can, when I saw a South Vietnamese soldier walking toward us. Suddenly he turned around and ran back. It was about the time I sat up and said "Huh" that the first mortar round hit in front of the helicopter, blowing all the Plexiglas out of the windows. We tried to take off and succeeded in getting off the ground when another and then another round hit. Somehow the helicopter flipped upside down and we mowed the grass with our main rotor blade. In other words, we crashed. Hard.

Doing a 180 at 60

I was knocked unconscious. The strange thing about being out is that you have absolutely no idea how long you were out. And when you come to, your brain has to reboot. Questions come in rapid succession.

Who am I?

Easy answer: John.

Where am I?

That's a little more difficult. Let's see. I'm in the Army, yeah. And I'm in Vietnam, that's better. Oh yeah, I'm in a helicopter. And, oh shit! We just crashed. WeJustCrashed. WEJUSTCRASHED.

It kind of just picked up speed from there. As it all came rushing back, I remembered that my helicopter was stuffed full of ammunition and jet fuel. If I didn't get my ass out of there, I was going to end up a crispy critter. That is, if there were enough parts of my blown-up body left to burn.

When I tried to get out of the helicopter, I found I couldn't. I still had my seat belt on. I released my seat belt and realized for the first time that I was upside down. Of course, the way I figured out that pretty important fact was that I landed on my head.

You know how you look around to see if anyone is watching when you do something dumb? I swear, here I was in the middle of a life and death catastrophe, and that's exactly what I did. I looked around.

No one saw me, though, because the helicopter had rolled partially toward my side.

I found a little crack of daylight, squeezed through, and stood up to run. But I had a bad case of the woozies, and for some reason my foot wouldn't hold me. So I crawled as fast as I could to get away from the helicopter before it blew up. And then, suddenly, some hands came out of the ground and pulled me into a foxhole I didn't even see. They started searching for holes in my body, and I pointed to my right leg, knowing something wasn't right even though I didn't feel any pain yet.

After some time, the South Vietnamese soldiers helped me out of their foxhole and dragged me, half hobbling, to a bunker on the other side of the hill, where I joined up with the rest of my crew. It seemed I was hurt the worst, with shrapnel wounds to my legs and a badly broken right foot with bones sticking out. I don't know how long we waited for a medevac helicopter, but eventually one sneaked in and got us out.

A few days later I was in Japan awaiting transfer back to the United States and read in the *Stars and Stripes* that the base where I was wounded was overrun. The soldiers who saved me were forced to retreat into the jungles. (This battle is chronicled in the book *Into Laos, Dewey Canyon II Lam Son 719* by Keith Nolan.)

I was only in Japan a short time before they loaded my stretcher into the back of a C141 with a giant, red cross on its tail and flew me back to the world (which is what we called the United States when we were over there). I got an early out (honorable discharge) and was back on the streets in 1972, not quite twenty-one years old.

This could have been the end of my flying dreams, because with my screwed up foot, I could no longer get into the helicopter flying program in the Army. But by now you know me better than that. Ever resilient, I bought my first book on how to be a pilot a while later.

But it seems it's always the same old story: got time but no money, or got money but no time. After a nine-year delay, I started my first official flying lesson at thirty-one years old. I actually made it through two lessons before I dislocated my right wrist in a work accident. By the time it was healed and I was ready to fly again, they closed the airport in Scotts Valley, California.

Four more years went flashing by, and in 1986 my friend Ken took me flying. I told him I didn't have a license, and he told me he didn't care. "Aim for that mountain peak," he said, and made me do most of the flying. He called me a week later and told me where I could buy an airplane really cheap.

"I don't have a license," I reminded him.

"That's the beauty of it," he said. "Once you own your own plane, all you do is hire an instructor and away you go."

Forever impulsive and loving a good deal for less than five grand, I bought a Piper Tomahawk that I later learned pilots call a "Traumahawk." I hired an instructor and soloed for the first time. I was thirty-six years old.

But wait, there's more (like the guy on TV says). I had my own business back then and was truly busy, busy, busy. Once again I found myself falling into the "got money, no time" trap. I was so busy I didn't have time for the ground school portion so I just kept flying on my student license. After awhile we had a brand new shiny daughter, so I sold the plane and moved to the mountains to raise some country kids.

In the early 1980s, I read a book on goal setting. I bought a good notebook and sat down and wrote out forty-one goals. I wasn't supposed to value judge them—like whether it's remotely possible to accomplish or not—just list them. I screwed up right off the bat when I wrote down that I wanted to buy a Mooney (a brand of single-engine, fast airplanes) for my first goal. I decided I'd better finish my pilot's license first, and buying the Mooney became my number two goal. I wrote my goals and had been crossing them off for many years.

In 1993 I took my goal book out and was disgusted about something and thought, "This is stupid. I'm never going to get my pilot's license." With my pen poised directly above it, I started to X it out of my life. But somehow I just couldn't do it. Instead I had a big talk with myself and said, "It's now or never!"

It was a busy time of life (again), so I made myself get up an hour early to study every morning. I made myself drive fifty miles to the closest airport and begin flying again. I did it the way I've always made myself do something, by putting one foot in front of the other.

Within five months, two weeks before my 43rd birthday, in the great and wonderful year of our Lord 1993, I passed my private pilot's test and was licensed. It was twenty years after buying my first book on flying. Strange, but after all that time you'd think I would have headed to the bar and got really sloshed, but by this time maturity had somehow kicked in. I felt a deeper, more complete satisfaction than I had ever thought possible.

Getting my pilot's license was the most tenacious thing I have ever done—well, that and reading *Zen and the Art of Motorcycle Maintenance*. Truth is, I started each about the same time and finished them somewhat together.

I've had some good flying times since that day and I got checked out again when I was sixty, after not flying for many long years. I must have been in pretty good health because I went to the flight surgeon and passed my physical. And I didn't even study.

Many people may not be aware of this, but once you have a pilot's license it's always active. However, one of the stipulations is that you have to pass your medical exam for it to be legal. And once you turn sixty, this is an annual requirement.

I once again had my class three medical, which allowed me to begin flying airplanes again. Look at what a simple easy sentence that is. Like you just show up and rent an airplane (if you don't own one) and off you soar into the wild blue yonder.

My redo was not so much a memorable flight as it was comfortable, like being with a long-lost friend.

Throughout the years I owned three other airplanes besides the Tomahawk, including a Mooney. Oh, yes. Dreams that become goals do become real. It happens all the time. I just never figured there would be such a long time gap in between.

* * *

Here's a strange truth for you. I bought *Zen and the Art of Motorcycle Maintenance* when I was twenty-three. If you know the book, you know it's not about fixing your motorcycle. (I didn't know that when I bought it.) I picked it up and put it down many times. The same year I passed my pilot's test, I began reading the book every morning in my new habit of quiet time, and after almost twenty years I finally finished it.

I've since reread the book many times and think, perhaps, that it is my favorite book ever. If you have read the book, you know the ending. If not, I'm not going to be the spoiler.

In a side note, the author's real-life son, Chris Pirsig, was only two weeks away from his 23rd birthday when he was murdered. Even though I never met him in real life, I felt his presence throughout the book, perhaps even more than if he were still alive. It seems to me, if any of us were to receive wings and fly, he would be at the top of the list.

He never made it to sixty.

13

The Thrill of Victory

By now you may have figured out that I don't have much fear of heights, or really anything. I'm not sure where it all started, but just maybe it came from my first time skiing.

It was in the winter of 1961 and I was ten years old. Back then we all watched the *Wide World of Sports*, with its famous introduction featuring "the thrill of victory and the agony of defeat." It always looked so easy, with the minor exception of some dude crashing off the ski-jump ramp and the other skiers crashing some of the time. It's amazing what you're willing to overlook when you really want to do something.

My dad had a pair of skis hanging up on the garage wall. To this day, I have never seen a pair of skis like them. Instead of any kind of bindings, they had a big fiberglass horseshoe-looking strap thingy that you slid your galoshes into.

You remember galoshes, right? They were big rubber boots that you crammed your shoes into, to keep them dry. And what was up with that weird buckle thing on the front that always hurt your fingers, especially when they were partially frozen? Oops, I did it again (a detour).

My dad's skis were probably cross-country skis, not the downhill kind, but when you're ten and it looks so easy, why wouldn't you try? I went down to the golf course and up the biggest hill I could find. I visited the golf course earlier this year, and the hills didn't look so big anymore, but when you're a ten-year-old squirt, they look enormous. Trust me on this, it's all about perspective. At ten, I thought those hills were as high as any mountain I've ever skied down since. And the feelings I had back then on that small slope are the same that I experience now.

There I was at ten years old, looking down the hill, skis dangling over the edge. From somewhere (probably the same place where it looked so easy), I found the courage and off I went. Thank God I had no ski poles with which to impale myself. After fifteen or twenty feet of pure ecstasy, I crashed. That was followed by thirty or forty feet of bouncing, rolling, flipping, and flopping. When I got up, I was at the bottom of the hill, looking like a miniature abominable snowman—make that snowboy—because back then we didn't have ski clothing that repels the snow.

You've probably guessed it, but right back up I went and did it over and over, again and again, until I finally made it all the way down without falling. And that was the precise time I realized that in all my "but it looks so easy" scenarios, I never thought about how to stop, except by crashing. I probably looked a lot like "the agony of defeat" dude.

That was the only time I skied, until my close friend Billy said, "Hey, John, let's go skiing. Oh don't worry, I'll teach you. It's really easy." The year was 1976, and I was nearly twenty-five.

Since that time I've had the skiing bug and have skied many times. It was a huge factor in my moving up to the mountains and teaching my kids, who were just little tykes, not to be afraid of dangling their skis over the edge and pushing off...of anything.

April 2005 was last time I went skiing. I had some medical issues two weeks after that and it put me on the shelf for a long time. After reading about all the stuff I've done, it seems strange to tell you I had colon surgery from something completely unrelated to sports.

Doing a 180 at 60

On April 16, 2012 a couple weeks before my 61st birthday, I went up to Kirkwood Ski resort and went sliding down the hills again with two boards attached to my feet. I learned a long time ago that the only thing that can get you in ski shape is skiing. Neither biking nor running (nor anything else) helps get you back in shape. I started on the bunny slopes and quickly progressed, tiring after many black diamond runs.

This was fine, because one of my favorite things about skiing is going into the bar and drinking winter ale afterward. And it was while doing just that I toasted one of the friends I hadn't thought of in a while.

***

Kim was a pretty girl in her twenties. We met when she worked in an office below mine and would come up to use our copy machine occasionally. The picture of health, she took some time off to have a mole removed from her back.

Three of us took her skiing for the last time in April 1991, and a very short time later (just over a month) she died of melanoma cancer. She never told any of us she had cancer, so none of us saw it coming.

She never made it to sixty.

14

If Your Friend Jumped Off a Bridge...

In some respects, bungee jumping and snow skiing are related. At first you might think they have nothing in common. And then you'd realize that for each of those activities you just ready-set-go and thrust yourself into the air. Standing at the edge of the bridge or tower is the same feeling I get in the pit of my stomach as when I look at my ski tips dangling over the edge of a really steep cliff. The difference is in the equipment. With skiing, you just push off with your poles to start the exhilarating, heart-pounding descent. When you dive off a bridge, not into the water but to dangle about in midair, there had better be a bungee cord—or to be more precise four of them—attached.

My first bungee experience was in 1994, when I was down in Florida visiting my brother-in-law Johnny. I gathered up my nephew and cousin and we went to the local arcade where they had a tower for bungee jumping. It was great fun.

When I climbed on the Internet to find someone to bungee with this time around, I was shocked that right here in my own little home town lives one of the first American pioneers of bungee jumping. And he was organizing a jump in just a few short weeks.

As it happened, we had booked a cruise to Mexico that ended in Long Beach, California, on Friday. The jump was scheduled for the following day early in the morning, way up in Northern California.

If you've been on a cruise, you know the ship is pretty neat and tidy, and the service is great. So you can imagine the culture shock of driving for twelve hours and ending up in a fleabag motel where I felt compelled to sleep with my pistol by my hand. I was surprised and delighted when I woke up in the morning and the whole car was still there.

My excitement continued to build as we drove an hour to a bridge that was one hundred seventy feet above a wild river. A few minutes later, the truck arrived with the other cars following. In no time at all, they had a platform hanging out from the bridge with the bungee outfit tied off, looking for the first victim, or rather volunteer.

Are you getting the sense that this was not a real professional organization? But once again, sometimes the not-so-well-scripted events turned out to be the best-est of the best. The first guy to jump told me he was so scared of heights he started bungee jumping just to cure himself, and he went off flawlessly. I never thought to ask him if a psychiatrist wrote a prescription or if he just figured it out for himself. The next girl had on her six-inch, crystal, pole-dancing, high-heeled shoes. And she did a marvelous jump.

I was next and I stood on the platform beyond the edge of the bridge, looking over the rim of the world. Or so it seemed. After I yelled a loud "Airborne" that echoed throughout the canyon, I dove straight out. If there had been an Olympic judge present, he surely would have given me a 10.0 or maybe 9.9 on a scale of 10. You can see my jump on JohnRTakacs.com.

The difference between bungee jumping and sky-diving is that you know for sure you're falling. You can see the bridge pass under you, and the trees on the river banks whiz by. The river is not coming up to meet you, but it looks like you're going to crash right into it until ... boing ... the bungee stretches out and you immediately begin heading back up in the opposite direction. You get to the apex of the return just below the bridge and once again fall right back down. You bounce a few more times until finally you stop and are suspended under the bridge, rather like a spider on a web. Then your fellow jumpers grab a line and triumphantly haul you back up.

Holy super cow, what a thrill!

And that would be the end of this story except for Katy. Katy's a good-looking, well-built, twenty-something (the preceding description was approved by my sweet girl), and she wanted to be thrown off the bridge. So four of us picked her up over our heads and at the count of three began shuffling forward. When we got to the guard rail, we threw her out into the raw air. And did she ever scream.

After she stopped bouncing, we pulled her back up. We found out she was an experienced bungee jumper, but never had the control of when to jump wrested from her. Being helplessly thrown from a bridge was like nothing she had ever felt before.

Now for the other part, which is: what I felt. If you've been divorced, I imagine you can relate to this. I think I always wanted to throw my ex off the bridge, at least figuratively. And when I threw little sweet Katy off, it was like fireworks going off inside. I just couldn't stop talking. I talked on and on until someone got a text alert, and we all scrambled off the bridge and stowed the bungee stuff away.

Right after the sheriff's car passed by, I found out that jumping off a bridge in California is just technically—or was it just slightly—against the law. Just like throwing your ex off. Talk about a no-funner state. I hope you realize that was all in jest, especially if you're divorced.

The video of my jump is posted on the website.

* * *

Let's go back to my first bungee jumping experience. I didn't mention that the reason I was in Florida in 1994 was that my brother-in-law Johnny was sick with cancer at the time. Taking the kids to the bungee tower was intended to help take their minds off their sorrow for a brief time. And maybe it was a great stress reliever for all of us who helplessly watched Johnny die of pancreatic cancer through the next few weeks.

When I tell you I have high emotional memories attached to those bungee days, I think you can now understand why.

Johnny was fifty-six years old.

He never made it to sixty.

15

Gentlemen, Start Your Engines

My friend Randy had a horse when we were growing up. I rode that mean son of a biscuit when I was a teenager. That dang horse would gently trot you down to the farthest corner of the property and then go into a gallop. While you were bouncing all around, he would then perform an emergency stop, putting his head down at the same time. Since we rode bareback, we would go sliding down his neck, crashing into the ground, and releasing the reins. The horse would then just trot back to his stall as if nothing had happened while we walked back, grumbling the whole way. (I rented a horse in my sixtieth year and had a nice mountain ride. A very pleasant redo instead of bitchin' and moaning.)

And that's one reason why my first and best love has always been motorcycles, especially dirt bikes.

Doing a 180 at 60

When you're done, you just put them away. Don't have to feed them. Don't have to clean up after them. Don't have to have this big confrontation with them when they want to go this way and you want to go the other. But wait a minute, sometimes the bike does want to go one way and you go the other. And come to think of it, you do have to wash it once in a while, like right after a race or something real muddy. As far as feeding the bike, it requires very little gas but lots of bucks for tires, helmets, gloves, boots, jerseys, shoulder pads, and maintenance. And the list goes on and on.

Golfing, bicycling, running, and swimming are all things I've done a lot of, but dirt bikes, without a doubt, have been my life's great love, as far as sports and activities are concerned.

I started riding the old scooter (that I wrote about in Chapter 4) long ago, and progressed to racing competitively after I got out of the Army in 1972, at the age of twenty-one. Two years later I discovered motocross racing and shortly after, I got involved in organized American Motorcycle Association (AMA) racing. Back in those days, much of motorcycle racing was just getting your bike to last long enough to get through the race intact.

Through the years, I've broken a set of handlebars, had my seat come off, lost my front sprocket, and—in my first big desert race—had a flat rear tire that I rode on for almost forty miles before it finally came off the rim. That didn't stop me, because I cut it off with a pair of side cutters and knife I carried in my tool kit. I put the tire and tube around my neck and rode into the pit where my pit crew put on a new tire that allowed me to finish the race. It was a great time and I did well in those years, becoming an expert or A-class racer.

In 1977 while leading in the Indiana State Motocross Championship, my rear brake broke. I had such a commanding lead that I held off the competition for many laps, until I was passed by four other riders and finished fifth overall. It was the best race I ever rode, going so fast without the benefit of being able to stop.

I took many firsts throughout the years, but some races—that were difficult either mechanically or due to weather (or both)—stand out more than others. In 1995, right before I turned forty-four, I entered the AMA National Hare Scrambles Championship and finished 4th nationally in my class, after missing the last two races when my transmission broke a main shaft and exited through the bottom of the motor.

Doing a 180 at 60

You may be wondering if I have ever been hurt doing any of these things? Oh, yes! I've had a few mishaps. Okay, I've had a bunch of injuries in my past. However, that's not the real issue. The better question would be, how do I feel now? The truth is, I have two things bothering me now. My left ankle has a strained ligament from too much golfing last year. And my left wrist that I'd never hurt badly enough to see a doctor about when I was younger now somehow has cartilage damage. An orthopedic doctor told me nothing can be done about it.

But I don't believe that.

The following paragraphs explain why.

One of the things that happened to me before I was thirty was tearing up my right knee while playing football. I had a completely torn posterior cruciate ligament (PCL), which was missed at the initial, totally incorrect, diagnosis in the emergency room. Later, when it didn't heal, I sought out a knee specialist. The knee doctor was the football and hockey specialist for Notre Dame. He told me my injury was rare as a football injury but a common hockey injury. It had to happen with the knee bent at a ninety-degree angle while striking the knee straight on, which is what happened when I dove for a tackle.

The doctor also told me it was too late for surgery. He recommended that I buy a bicycle and ride the wheels off. In other words, build the muscle around the knee to take up the slack. I had a lot of slack, being able to push and pull my lower leg an inch or more. He said to keep checking in over the years in case any advances in modern medicine became viable for me.

I did see doctors throughout the years and had a couple of MRI's showing that nothing had changed, until the year 2000. At forty-nine I was running a lot, and coming down a hill one day, I suddenly had some big-time pain. It was so bad I ended up limping back a couple of miles. Once again, it wasn't healing, so I made an appointment with another orthopedic doc. An MRI showed that I had a torn a meniscus in the same knee. We discussed the MRI, and later on I had arthroscopic surgery. But while we were talking about the injury, I asked about the torn PCL. The doc told me it was not torn all the way through, but was hanging by a thread.

That was weird but I let it go, thinking maybe the other doctors were just rounding off or something like that. Well, lo and behold, nine years later I went in again for the same knee, which was hurting in a completely different spot: directly in front, under the knee cap. A totally different orthopedic doc told me, while looking at the new MRI, that it looked like I had a defect, as my knee cap had some kind of weird wear pattern. I told him that was probably because of the excessive slop from my torn PCL. He checked the MRI again and then informed me I didn't have a torn PCL.

Remembering the rounding-off theory I said, "Oh yeah, it's hanging by a thread."

He said, "No the ligament is fine."

The argument was just starting when I had him check my old MRIs. He compared them and in a conversational voice said, "It has totally re-grown. I guess you're a medical miracle."

I wanted to shout out loud, "Me, a medical miracle!"

Instead, I asked how that could be.

So many different doctors had accused me of abusing my own body—sometimes silently, with the rolling of eyes or shaking of a head, and sometimes more emphatically—when all I was trying to do was live…excitingly. I have much to say on this, and it's only a chapter away.

Meanwhile, there seemed to be a shift going on in the doctor world, and this doctor was more enlightened than most. He asked about supplements I was taking, and I informed him that I started taking glucosamine seventeen years before, after I'd read some articles touting it.

I've also read more recent studies saying glucosamine doesn't work. I know that we are all different, and I wasn't one of the people in the more recent studies that were funded by the pharmaceutical companies. I also know that my ligament was totally severed and completely healed itself after I started taking glucosamine.

So what's up with this long dissertation? I take many supplements each day, but no prescription medications. I don't even take aspirin. I've had many broken bones throughout the years, but don't seem to have any arthritis in my body. Just about everyone (from well-meaning friends to different doctors) has warned me about arthritis. The common phrase, I believe, was "when you get old..."

My whole point in telling this story is to point out that I discovered alternative medicine while racing motorcycles in the nineties. There is more than one school of thought (more than the pill pushers) when it comes to your health. How come a drug doesn't work on each of us the same way, but instead gives different results? It helps one person, another stays the same, and another it kills. And what about side effects? Because we are all different, you just might respond better to chiropractic, acupuncture, massage, Ayurvedic, or my favorite: Active ReleaseTechnique.

I have a room in my basement with four dirt bikes, which I hadn't ridden for at least four years at the time of this writing. That changed with my last redo, since I saved the best for last. Another reason I saved it for last was that motorcycling is the most difficult and the most dangerous of all my redo attempts. If I hurt myself on this activity, I wouldn't have a chance to do any of the others.

I lived for the times when my motorcycle and I became one. It's like slow motion and I'm in a time chamber knowing how everything moves around me. If there weren't so many busy things going on at the same time, I swear I'd see my own breath. I'm so much in the zone everything becomes crystal clear, almost like I'd done it a million times before. And there is no conscious thought.

It's like when you come to the top of a jump and the back wheel unexpectedly hits a rock and jumps sideways. While you're in the air, you turn the bike to land exactly like it's supposed to land. It's all done so quickly your mind doesn't even have time to say, "Oh, crap!" The thrill that comes from racing is probably all about that one oh-crap second when life in all its essence is well lived.

I loved slipping and sliding through the woods and mountains, and even the deserts, as fast as the bike would go, wide open. The need for speed is the feeling that kept me racing for more than thirty years.

My intention was to go motorcycle racing as the last item on my redo list. But instead I decided to go up into the mountains one last time to do what I enjoyed maybe more than racing. And that was just plain old riding, what we call cow trailing. Somehow it turned out to be more fitting, probably because when I first started riding, I rode in the woods and fields long before I hit the racetrack.

Like so many other times in this season of redoing, it wasn't my last time to ride. After one ride, the bug bit me again, and I now go all the time. As hard as it may be to believe, it's just as good now as it ever was. Maybe I'm not quite as good, but the rides are, and once again I seem to have come full circle.

* * *

When I was in my twenties I rode almost every day, practicing hour after hour. I raced every weekend in season and was constantly working on my bikes to keep them in tiptop shape. As we said back then, I ate, drank, and dreamt motorcycles. I wanted to turn pro, but once again life had gotten in the way.

Doing a 180 at 60

One of the guys I spent some time with was a young kid named Max. Where I had to work hard on my form and technique, he was a natural. He could take any motorcycle, from a dirt bike to a big street bike, and ride a wheelie for a half mile or more. It was as if he had a gyrostabilizer in his head.

There is no doubt he would have been a great professional. *Would have* are the key words in that sentence, because while passing another car in his Pinto wagon he was tragically killed.

It never made any sense to me. He had such great instincts and coordination. He was nineteen years old.

He never made it to sixty.

16

The Last Word

When I started my list of things I wanted to do again, it had thirty-three items on it. That list grew to forty-something. And then I thought how clever it would be to put sixty activities on the list. You know, it just seemed right.

Once I started on the list, I was surprised by how much time it took to get into the kind of shape required to do many of the things. There were a few things on my list that I knew I probably couldn't (or wouldn't be allowed to) do, like tackle football and pole vaulting, for instance. It's not that I wouldn't be able to do them. It's just that finding someone or some team that would allow me to try out was not likely.

Recently I was in a yoga class, another redo, and the instructor or yogi master or whatever they are called, pointed me out as an example. For a change, I was the good example. One of the students objected, "Yeah, but he's an athlete."

I couldn't help but wonder: where was this guy when I was an overly fat writer, totally out of shape and struggling with my weight? Nevertheless, it was the first time in this century that I thought of myself as an athlete.

Most of us are similar in thinking if only I were _____ (fill in the blank: taller, faster, stronger, bigger, slimmer, the list is endless), I could have been a great athlete. I'm 5'10" and weigh about 185 pounds. I was taller when I was younger, I'm sure.

The next sentence is possibly the weirdest statement in this book. Here goes: perhaps I have had the perfect athletic body all this time. When I look around, there are virtually no (or at best very few) men in my age group doing anything physically demanding.

Look at that statement again and then look around. I'm talking about former professional athletes, also. I am not claiming to be a great athlete. I'm probably slightly above average—at best—talent-wise, but world class in desire. I think that might be the great secret.

So what's it all about?

Life. Breath. Belief.

I'll bet you knew all along that this subject was going to be coming up. None of us can hold off the inevitable. No one gets out of this alive. No religion here, I'm talking physically. Almost all sane people have the same goal, to live a long time. And I mean really live, not just exist. It's about quality of life.

Ask around. None of us want to spend our last days in a nursing home. Is that because we view that as merely existing and not truly living? If I were to die tomorrow while on a bicycle ride, instead of dying twenty years from now after a slow boring life, that would constitute for me a great life. This does not mean that I am ready to die. As Kenny Chesney sings, "Everybody want to go to Heaven, but nobody want to go now."

How about you?

What about the quality of your life?

My mom, who is now ninety-four and hasn't a mean bone in her body, was struggling to say something nice about a man who had recently died. After a few attempts she said, "You know, he was a really good TV watcher."

Pffftt! A watcher: someone who sees other people's glory and has none of his or her own. In using the term "glory," I don't mean winning an Ironman Triathlon, a marathon, or something equally noble. The glory comes from within when you simply finish something difficult and worthy.

Doing a 180 at 60

How much different would your life be if you could just get motivated, get out of that easy chair, and begin going back and doing some fun things again?

My advice? Talk to your doctor, then start slow.

For most of my life I've had people shaking their heads and telling me what's not possible. Sometimes they tell me, "Yeah, that's easy for you, but I can't because _____ (fill in the blank, once again).

Here's the real deal. Many of our physical problems revolve around our weight. If not our weight, it's probably the side effects of the medicine that's become a crutch for us. I know that's a tough statement, but that was my story.

I told a friend in Florida the same thing I'm writing here: a swimming pool is a great place to begin your cardio exercise again. The water doesn't know you're overweight, and once you're in the water, neither does your body.

I encourage you to become a student again: get online and read, take a class and study, ask your doctor, find out everything there is to know about your health issues.

Most of all, be open minded. But don't look for advice from other victims. Instead look for the exception that you can then become.

I was on a radio talk show a few months back, and the host and I talked about the people we see in grocery stores riding around on electric scooters. Almost all are overweight. I can't help but think that if they walked more they wouldn't be as overweight, but because they are so overweight they can't walk. It's a true Catch-22.

I started the book with the words: I. Was. Wrong. Once again I remind you of that. The sports and activities that built such a rich and rewarding life for you and for me aren't just for the young. I've proven that. I don't know why I stopped doing so many of the things I truly loved doing. I really don't have a clue. I don't know why I thought I had to live life as if there were some kind of mandatory profile neatly written up, telling me how old people were supposed to act.

And once again, at what age are we old? With obesity running rampant it could probably be argued that some teens are living in sixty-year-old bodies.

I really don't like to hear people say, "Getting old is a bitch." Because what's the alternative? What's the other choice? Dying.

If I were to get religious, I would tell you that fear is the devil's number one weapon." Please don't let fear stop you.

Doing a 180 at 60

I do know that it wasn't hard to change things around. And yes, I'm enjoying the hell out of my life now.

More than anything, I want you to come join me. No, I don't mean you have to sign up for Ironman events, go skydiving, or even motorcycle racing. But you could start by parking farther away from the gym when you work out, taking walks in the evening, and saying no to that fast food or piece of pie.

Remember, sixty is the youth of old age, and a 180 (or You-Turn) can be just ahead for you.

180 at 60 Redo List

☑	Scuba Diving	☑	Swim One Mile
☐	Long Bicycle Tour	☐	Fishing
☑	Golfing	☐	Skeet Shooting
☑	Skydiving	☑	Weightlifting
☑	Flying	☐	Volleyball
☑	Motorcycle Tour	☐	Croquet
☐	Abalone Diving	☐	Badminton
☐	Water Skiing	☑	Horseback Riding
☑	Snow Skiing	☑	Bungee Jumping
☑	Day Hiking	☑	Zip Line
☑	Dirt Bike Riding	☑	Rappelling
☑	Racquetball	☐	Roller Skating
☑	Basketball	☐	Inline Skating
☐	Baseball	☐	Ice Skating
☐	Football	☐	Hockey
☐	Tennis	☑	Spelunking
☑	Ping Pong	☐	Pole Vaulting
☑	Bowling	☐	High Jumping
☑	Pool	☐	Karate
☑	Horseshoes	☑	Dancing
☐	Snowmobiling	☐	Soccer
☑	Jet Skiing	☐	Snowshoeing
☑	Canoeing	☑	Handball
☑	Kayaking	☑	Yoga
☑	Whitewater Rafting	☐	Archery
☑	Diving off Rocks	☐	Trampoline
☑	Diving off Rope Swing	☐	Backpacking
☑	Triathlon	☑	Rock Climbing
☑	Wake Board	☑	Mountain Biking
☑	Run a Marathon	☑	Write Nonfiction Book

Acknowledgments

I didn't include this story in the book so here's the last one.

In December 2015, my best friend—the sweet girl referenced in this book, now my wonderful wife—and I entered the California International Marathon. It was a first for both of us. For many miles we would hold hands as we ran, and I say to this day it was a very romantic time.

Shows how weird I am, when in fact I was huffing and puffing along, first in the rain and then in almost total exhaustion. There's a point when you get so tired, though, that your brain ceases its endless chattering. At that point a calming wall of silence envelopes you, and I would say that is as close to heaven or nirvana as anyone could ever hope to attain on earth.

Most do not know how time consuming training for an Ironman is: six days a week, many of them from early morning until past ten at night. If you add to that an author's lifestyle (which tends to be solitary and often spent looking at the wall while inside your head you are a million miles away) you will understand why this book is dedicated to my so-very-patient, sweet girl. Monika.

About John Takacs

John Takacs is the author of the award-winning novel *The Take-Us*, an adventure thriller about an inventor who modifies a car to run without gasoline, which results in the awakening of Middle Eastern sleeper cells across the continent.

In 1971 John was combat wounded while serving with the famed 101st Airborne Division in Vietnam. The Huey helicopter he was in was shot down. John was put on a medevac plane to Japan, and a few days later was off-loaded on a stretcher at Great Lakes Naval Hospital where he was awarded the Purple Heart Medal.

Always the adventurist and outdoor enthusiast, John competed in the Ironman 70.3 World Championship in 2016 at the age of sixty-five. He lives with his wife Monika in Pioneer, California.

* * *

Visit John at his website, www.JohnRTakacs.com, for further information, photos, and videos of his journey.